Applying the Evidence: Clinical Trials in Diabetes

Published by Remedica

Commonwealth House, 1 New Oxford Street, London, WC1A 1NU, UK
Civic Opera Building, 20 N Wacker Drive, Suite 1642, Chicago, IL, USA

info@remedicabooks.com
www.remedicabooks.com
Tel: +44 (0)20 7759 2999
Fax: +44 (0)20 7759 2951

Publisher: Andrew Ward
Commissioning Editor: Philip Shaw
Editors: Catherine Harris, Carolyn Dunn and Anuradha Choudhury
Design and artwork: AS&K Skylight Creative Services
Production Manager: Mary Hughes
© 2005 Remedica

Remedica is a member of the AS&K Media Partnership.

ISBN-13: 978 1 850092 84 2
ISBN-10: 1 850092 84 2
British Library Cataloguing-in-Publication Data
A catalogue record for this book is available from the British Library.

Applying the Evidence: Clinical Trials in Diabetes

Anthony Barnett
Birmingham Heartlands Hospital
Birmingham, UK

Contents

Introduction

When I first started out in diabetes at Kings College Hospital, London, back in 1978, the emphasis of management related to blood glucose control. We were certainly aware that hypertension was an important risk factor for cardiovascular disease and that some diabetic patients also had abnormalities of their lipid profile; high blood pressure was commonly recognised and treated but there was a very small evidence base from trials in diabetic patients to guide such treatment, and none at all from the point of view of lipid management. We also screened for diabetic microvascular disease, particularly retinopathy, but we were only just starting to recognise the terrible rate of attrition from cardiovascular disease. Our therapeutic armamentarium was extremely limited and our evidence base for treatment very much anecdotal – and non-existent from the point of view of robust scientific study. How times have changed!

The last 20 years, and in particular the last 10 years, have seen a veritable explosion in the evidence base for the management of diabetes. Multiprofessional care has come into its own; we better understand the epidemiology of diabetes, and its complications and pathogenetic mechanisms are being identified. Robust scientific studies have been produced, new drugs have come on the scene and the evidence base for management is now outstanding. We at last recognise that type 2 diabetes, in particular, is a cardiovascular risk equivalent. We also recognise the importance of a multiprofessional approach to management, with the patient as the central character. Multiple cardiovascular risk factor intervention has become the norm. We are now also in the position to save vision, preserve renal function and (perhaps) prevent neuropathy.

A host of important studies has led to remarkable advances in diabetes care in recent years. In putting together this book on clinical trials in diabetes and how they have impacted on diabetes management, it has been extremely difficult to pick out the most important ones from the many thousands that have been published during that time. This is one author's attempt to do just that and I apologise to those investigators who have spent years adding to our knowledge base if their particular trial(s) has been omitted. I have, though, tried to select those trials that I believe have had the most important practical significance in advising clinicians on diabetes management best practice. Our readers will note that there is a particular emphasis on UKPDS, which many believe is the most important clinical trial ever produced in the field of type 2 diabetes.

1

One could also argue similarly for the Diabetes Control and Complications Trial in type 1 diabetes, although the magnitude of type 1 diabetes as a public health problem is dwarfed by the epidemic we now have in type 2 diabetes. There are, however, some extremely important landmark trials which are nothing to do with UKPDS and DCCT! I have tried to include as many of these as possible in this brief review.

I hope that the readership finds my selection of trials both appropriate and interesting, as well as informative in helping with clinical practice. In the commentary for each I have tried to provide some practical suggestions as to the implications of each trial, although it is important not to take each trial in isolation. Many of them complement each other and inform indirectly on practice.

I hope that our readers find this a useful, practical and highly readable book.

Professor Anthony Barnett, BSc (Hons), MD, FRCP
Professor of Medicine

Intensive Glucose Control

Intensive blood-glucose control with sulphonylureas or insulin compared with conventional treatment and risk of complications in patients with type 2 diabetes (UKPDS 33)

What does this trial tell us?

➤ Intensive blood-glucose control by either sulphonylureas or insulin substantially decreases the risk of microvascular complications, but not macrovascular disease, in patients with type 2 diabetes

➤ None of the drugs under investigation had an adverse effect on cardiovascular outcomes

Authors	UK Prospective Diabetes Study (UKPDS) Group
Reference	*Lancet* 1998;352:837–53
Objective	To compare the effects of intensive blood glucose control with either sulphonylurea or insulin and conventional treatment on the risk of microvascular and macrovascular complications in patients with type 2 diabetes
Drugs used	Insulin, chlorpropamide, glibenclamide, glipizide
Patients	3,867, with newly diagnosed type 2 diabetes, mean age 54 years
Outcomes	Three aggregate endpoints: any diabetes-related endpoint (sudden death, death from hyperglycaemia or hypoglycaemia, fatal or non-fatal myocardial infarction, angina, heart failure, stroke, renal failure, amputation of at least one digit, vitreous haemorrhage, retinopathy requiring photocoagulation, blindness in one eye, cataract extraction), diabetes-related death and all-cause mortality
Analysis	Intention to treat
Follow-up	10 years

Results

	Patients with clinical endpoints		Absolute risk events per 1,000 patient-years		Log rank P	RR for intensive policy
	Intensive (n=2,729)	Conventional (n=1,138)	Intensive	Conventional		
AGGREGATE ENDPOINTS						
Any diabetes-related endpoint	263	428	40.9	46.0	0.029	0.88 (0.79–0.99)
Diabetes-related deaths	285	129	10.4	11.5	0.34	0.90 (0.73–1.11)
All-cause mortality	489	213	17.9	18.9	0.44	0.94 (0.80–1.10)
SINGLE ENDPOINTS						
Death from peripheral vascular disease	2	8	0.1	0.3	0.12	0.26 (0.03–2.77)
Amputation	27	18	1.0	1.6	0.059	0.61 (0.28–1.33)
Death from renal disease	8	2	0.3	0.2	0.53	1.63 (0.21–12.49)
Renal failure	16	9	0.6	0.8	0.45	0.73 (0.25–2.14)
Retinal photocoagulation	207	117	7.9	11.0	0.0031	0.71 (0.53–0.96)
Vitreous haemorrhage	19	10	0.7	0.9	0.51	0.77 (0.28–2.11)
Blind in one eye	78	38	2.9	3.5	0.29	0.84 (0.51–1.40)
Cataract extraction	149	80	5.6	7.4	0.046	0.76 (0.53–1.08)

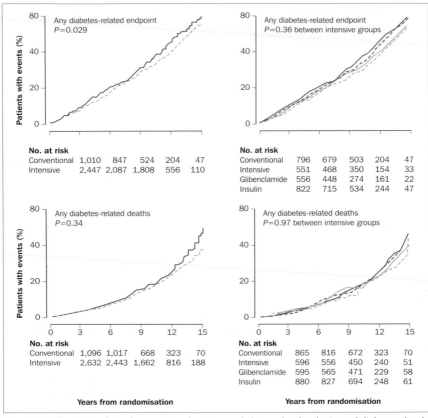

Figure 1. Kaplan-Meier plots of aggregate endpoints: any diabetes-related endpoint and diabetes-related death for conventional or intensive treatment, and by individual intensive therapy. Reproduced with permission from *The Lancet*.

Commentary

This study proved conclusively the value of "tight" diabetes control in prevention of long-term microvascular complications in type 2 diabetes, although interestingly no reduction in risk of macrovascular disease was demonstrated (reduction in risk of myocardial infarction almost reached clinical significance ($P<0.052$). This study has led to a range of national and international recommendations for target HbA_{1c} levels in type 2 diabetes, and – taken with other reports from the UKPDS programme – has led to major changes in diabetes practice.

The effect of intensive treatment of diabetes on the development and progression of long-term complications in insulin-dependent diabetes mellitus

What does this trial tell us?

➤ Intensive insulin therapy in patients with insulin-dependent diabetes delays the onset and slows the progression of diabetic retinopathy, nephropathy and neuropathy

➤ Because of the increased risk of hypoglycaemia, intensive therapy should be instituted with caution and frequent monitoring

Authors	The Diabetes Control and Complications Trial Research Group
Reference	*N Engl J Med* 1993;329:977–86
Objective	To determine whether intensive treatment with the goal of maintaining blood glucose concentrations close to the normal range could decrease the frequency of major microvascular and neurological complications
Methodology	Randomised controlled trial. Patients assigned to either: (a) intensive therapy with an external insulin pump or by three or four daily insulin injections, guided by frequent blood glucose monitoring; or (b) conventional therapy with once- or twice- daily insulin injections
Drugs used	Insulin, including mixed intermediate and rapid-acting insulins
Patients	1,441 patients, aged 13–39 years, with insulin-dependent diabetes: 726 with no retinopathy at baseline (the primary prevention cohort) and 715 with mild retinopathy (the secondary intervention cohort)
Outcomes	Retinopathy (as measured by fundal photography), urinary albumin excretion and clinical neuropathy
Analysis	Intention to treat
Follow-up	Mean 6.5 years

Results

Percentage risk reduction with intensive diabetes treatment compared with conventional therapy			
Complication	Primary prevention cohort	Secondary intervention cohort	Both cohorts combined
≥ 3-step sustained retinopathy	76 (P≤ 0.002)	54 (P≤ 0.002)	63 (P≤ 0.002)
Severe retinopathy	–	47 (P<0.04)	47 (P<0.04)
Microalbuminuria	34 (P<0.04)	43 (P≤ 0.002)	39 (P≤ 0.002)
Albuminuria	44	56 (P<0.04)	54 (P<0.04)
Clinical neuropathy at 5 years	69	57 (P≤ 0.002)	60 (P≤ 0.002)

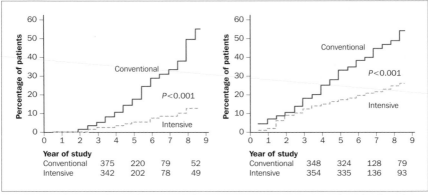

Figure 2. Cumulative incidence of a sustained change in retinopathy in patients with insulin-dependent diabetes receiving intensive or conventional therapy. (**Left**) Primary prevention cohort. (**Right**) Secondary intervention cohort. Reproduced with permission from the Massachusetts Medical Society.

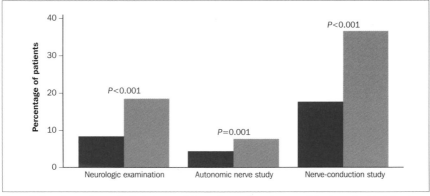

Figure 3. Prevalence of neurological abnormalities at 5 years in patients receiving intensive (dark bars) or conventional (pale bars) therapy. Reproduced with permission from the Massachusetts Medical Society.

Commentary

This landmark paper conclusively confirmed that intensive treatment of type 1 diabetes, leading to tightened diabetic control, is associated with a significantly reduced risk for the development and progression of microvascular complications. It has led to and supported a range of national and international guidelines on the glycaemic management of type 1 diabetes. It is also responsible, in part, for a multitude of studies looking at methods for intensification of insulin therapy and overall improvement in glycaemic control.

Effect of intensive blood-glucose control with metformin on complications in overweight patients with type 2 diabetes (UKPDS 34)

What does this trial tell us?

➤ Intensive blood glucose control with metformin appears to decrease the risk of diabetes-related endpoints in overweight diabetic patients

➤ The treatment is associated with less weight gain and fewer hypoglycaemic attacks than treatment with insulin and sulphonylureas

➤ Intensive glucose control with metformin might be the first-line choice of pharmacological therapy in these patients

Authors	UK Prospective Diabetes Study (UKPDS) Group
Reference	*Lancet* 1998;352:854–65
Objective	To determine whether intensive glucose control with metformin has any specific advantage or disadvantage over conventional treatment
Methodology	Randomised controlled trial of conventional treatment, mainly with diet alone, versus intensive blood glucose control with metformin, aiming for fasting plasma glucose (FPG) <6 mmol/L
Drugs used	Chlorpropamide, glibenclamide, insulin and metformin; dose according to FPG
Patients	1,704 overweight patients with newly diagnosed type 2 diabetes (FPG 6.1–15.0 mmol/L)
Outcomes	Primary outcome measures were time to first occurrence of any diabetes-related clinical endpoint (eg, renal failure, stroke), diabetes-related death and all-cause mortality. Secondary endpoints included myocardial infarction and stroke
Analysis	Intention to treat
Follow-up	Median 10.7 years

Results

Outcome	P for metformin versus other intensive treatment	Absolute risk (events per 1,000 patient-years)		Relative risk versus conventional treatment
		Metformin	Conventional	
Any diabetes-related endpoint	0.0034			
Metformin		29.8	43.8	0.68
Intensive		40.1	43.8	0.98
Diabetes-related death	0.11			
Metformin		7.5	12.7	0.58
Intensive		10.8	12.7	0.80
All-cause mortality	0.001			
Metformin		13.5	20.6	0.64
Intensive		18.9	20.6	0.52

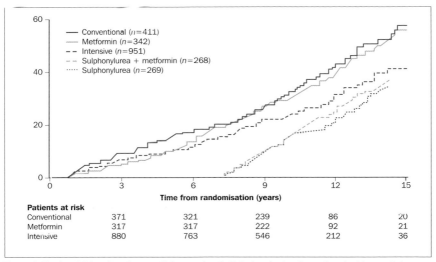

Figure 4. Kaplan–Meier plots for any diabetes-related clinical endpoint. Reproduced with permission from *The Lancet*.

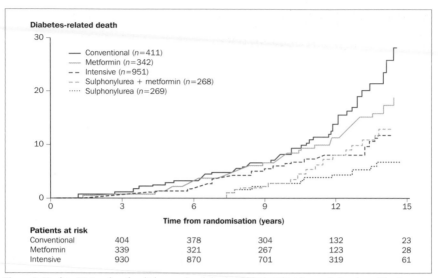

Figure 5. Kaplan–Meier plots for diabetes-related death. Reproduced with permission from *The Lancet*.

Commentary

Although UKPDS as a whole did not show evidence for cardiovascular protection in type 2 diabetes from tightened glycaemic control, the exception to this was in overweight patients prescribed metformin. The use of metformin was associated with a reduction of risk for any diabetes-related endpoint, diabetes-related death and all-cause mortality. This study proved beyond reasonable doubt that metformin should be the first-line pharmacotherapeutic treatment in the management of type 2 diabetes.

Quality of life in type 2 diabetic patients is affected by complications but not by intensive policies to improve blood glucose or blood pressure control (UKPDS 37)

What does this trial tell us?

➤ In patients with type 2 diabetes, quality of life (QOL) is affected by complications of the disease, but not by therapeutic policies shown to reduce the risk of complications

➤ It is uncertain whether frequent hypoglycaemic episodes affect QOL, or whether patients with certain personality traits report increased numbers of hypoglycaemic attacks

Authors	UK Prospective Diabetes Study (UKPDS) Group
Reference	*Diabetes Care* 1999;22:1125–36
Objective	To determine, in patients with type 2 diabetes, the effects on QOL of therapies for improving blood pressure (BP) control and diabetic complications, and for reducing hypoglycaemic episodes
Methodology	1. Two cross-sectional studies of patients enrolled in randomised controlled trials of: (a) intensive blood glucose control compared with conventional blood glucose control; and (b) a tight BP control policy (patients randomly allocated to either angiotensin-converting enzyme [ACE] inhibitors or beta-blockers) compared with less tight BP control (avoiding ACE inhibitors and beta-blockers)
	2. A longitudinal study of patients in a randomised controlled trial of intensive blood glucose control compared with conventional blood glucose control
	All patients, including controls, completed detailed QOL questionnaires
Patients	Respectively in the three trials: 2,431 (mean age 60 years), 3,104 (mean age 62 years) and 374 patients with type 2 diabetes (mean age 52 years); 122 non-diabetic control subjects (mean age 62 years)

Outcomes   Work satisfaction, mood state, cognitive failures (with relative's report), symptoms and general health (eg, mobility, pain)

Analysis   Intention to treat

Follow-up   6 years

Results

Effect of allocated therapies		
Both cross-sectional and longitudinal studies showed no effect of therapies on:		
1. mood 2. cognitive mistakes 3. symptoms 4. work satisfaction 5. general health		
Effect of complications (comparison of presence and absence of complications in preceding year)		
Macrovascular complications	Microvascular complications	Hypoglycaemic episodes (two or more in preceding year)
1. Worse general health ($P=0.0006-0.0012$)	1. More tension ($P=0.0082$)	1. More tension ($P=0.0023$)
2. More mobility problems ($P<0.0001$)	2. More mood disturbance ($P=0.0054$)	2. More mood disturbance ($P=0.0009$)
3. More problems with usual activities ($P=0.0023$)		3. Less work satisfaction ($P=0.0042$)
4. Reduced vigour ($P=0.0077$)		

Commentary

For years, many health professionals have been reluctant to intensify diabetes management in the mistaken belief that by withholding insulin, for example, they are in some way preserving the patient's QOL. Nothing could be further from the truth. This point is extremely well emphasised in this important study.

The authors looked at the effects on QOL of therapies for improving BP control and diabetic complications, and for reducing hypoglycaemic episodes. The main finding was that, in patients with type 2 diabetes, QOL is affected more by the complications of the disease than by the therapeutic treatment. The only caveat to this is where the treatment induces more frequent (particularly severe) hypoglycaemic episodes, which could have a negative effect on QOL.

Tight blood pressure control and risk of macrovascular and microvascular complications in type 2 diabetes (UKPDS 38)

What does this trial tell us?

➤ Tight blood pressure (BP) control using an angiotensin-converting enzyme inhibitor or beta-blocker in diabetic patients is successful, achieving a mean of 144/82 mm Hg in this study

➤ More than one antihypertensive might be required; 29% of the patients required three or more

➤ Fatal and non-fatal cardiovascular complications and deterioration in visual acuity are reduced by tight control of BP compared with less tight control

Authors	UK Prospective Diabetes Study (UKPDS) Group
Reference	*BMJ* 1998;317:703–13
Objective	To determine whether tight control of BP prevents macrovascular and microvascular complications in patients with type 2 diabetes
Methodology	Randomised controlled trial of tight BP control (aiming for <150/85 mm Hg) versus less tight control (aiming for <180/105 mm Hg)
Drugs used	Captopril, atenolol (for comparative effects see UKPDS 39, *BMJ* 1998;317:713–20)
Patients	1,148 hypertensive patients with type 2 diabetes, mean age 56 years, mean BP at entry 160/94 mm Hg. A total of 758 patients were allocated to tight BP control and 390 patients to less tight control
Outcomes	21 predefined clinical endpoints, including deaths related to diabetes, all-cause mortality, urinary albumin excretion and visual acuity
Analysis	Intention to treat
Follow-up	Median 8.4 years

Results

	Tight BP control	Less tight BP control
Mean BP (mm Hg)	144/82	154/87
Any diabetes-related endpoint (events per 1,000 patient-years)	50.9	67.4 (P<0.005, 24% relative risk reduction)
All-cause mortality (events per 1,000 patient-years)	22.4	27.2 (non-significant, P=0.17)
Myocardial infarction (events per 1,000 patient-years)	18.6	23.5 (non-significant, P=0.13)
Stroke (events per 1,000 patient-years)	6.5	11.6 (P<0.01, 44% relative risk reduction)
Microvascular disease (events per 1,000 patient-years)	12.0	19.2 (P<0.01, 37% relative risk reduction)
Retinopathy	47% reduction in the risk of a decrease in vision by three lines or more in both eyes (measured with an ETDRS chart) with tight BP control (P=0.004)	

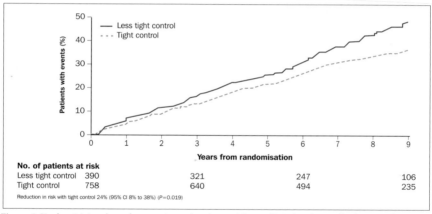

Figure 6. Kaplan–Meier plots of proportions of patients with any clinical endpoint, fatal or non-fatal, related to diabetes. CI: confidence interval. Reproduced with permission from the BMJ Publishing Group.

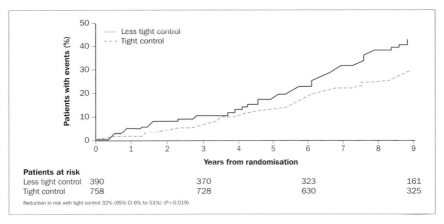

Figure 7. Kaplan–Meier plots of proportions of patients who die of disease related to diabetes (myocardial infarction, sudden death, stroke, peripheral vascular disease or renal failure). CI: confidence interval. Reproduced with permission from the BMJ Publishing Group.

Commentary

The objective of this substudy was to determine whether or not 'tight' control of BP prevented macrovascular complications in patients with type 2 diabetes. The mean achieved BP was significantly lower at 144/82 mm Hg in the 'tight' control group compared with 154/87 mm Hg in the 'less tight' control group ($P<0.0001$). This difference of 10/5 mm Hg was associated with significant reductions in macrovascular and microvascular events: all diabetes endpoints were significantly reduced by 24%, as was stroke (by 44%) and microvascular disease (by 37%). The reduction in microvascular complications was predominantly attributable to a reduced risk of retinopathy and its progression.

The study reinforced the view that control of BP in diabetic patients is of the utmost importance in determining long-term outcome. BP should be regularly monitored in patients with diabetes and aggressively treated to goal in order to minimise later complications. This might require a combination of several antihypertensive drugs. The authors suggested that definitions of BP used in guidelines – including terms such as 'fair' and 'acceptable' – should be reviewed in light of the results of this study.

Effect of intensive therapy on the microvascular complications of type 1 diabetes mellitus

What does this trial tell us?

➤ In type 1 diabetes, intensive treatment significantly reduces the risks of retinopathy, nephropathy and neuropathy compared with conventional treatment

➤ Absolute risks of retinopathy and nephropathy are proportional to the mean HbA_{1c} level

➤ The benefits of intensive treatment extend well beyond the period of its most intensive implementation

Authors	The Writing Team for the Diabetes Control and Complications Trial (DCCT)/Epidemiology of Diabetes Interventions and Complications Research Group
Reference	*JAMA* 2002;287:2563–9
Objective	To investigate the effects of intensive treatment on the microvascular complications of type 1 diabetes
Methodology	1. Randomised controlled clinical trial comparing intensive and conventional treatment
	2. Observational follow-up, following early termination of controlled trial after benefits of intensive treatment were deemed incontrovertible
Drugs used	Insulin by multiple (3–4) daily injections or continuous infusion in intensive group; conventional treatment with 1–2 daily injections in conventional group
Patients	1,441 patients, aged 13–39 years, with type 1 diabetes and no severe microvascular complications
Outcomes	Retinopathy, nephropathy and neuropathy
Analysis	Intention to treat
Follow-up	Controlled clinical trial: 6.5 years; observational follow-up: 7 years

Results

Incidence of worsening of complications between end of controlled trial and after 4 years of observational study			
	Patients who progressed, n (%)	Adjusted odds reduction, %	P value
Retinal change			
3-step progression from no retinopathy			
Conventional therapy	18 (16)		
Intensive therapy	11 (6)	66	0.006
Severe non-proliferative retinopathy or worse			
Conventional therapy	53 (10)		
Intensive therapy	11 (2)	76	<0.001
Proliferative retinopathy			
Conventional therapy	48 (9)		
Intensive therapy	10 (2)	74	<0.001
Clinically significant macular oedema			
Conventional therapy	45 (8)		
Intensive therapy	9 (2)	77	<0.001
Renal change			
Microalbuminuria			
Conventional therapy	63 (11)		
Intensive therapy	31 (5)	53	0.002
Albuminuria			
Conventional therapy	33 (5)		
Intensive therapy	4 (1)	86	<0.001

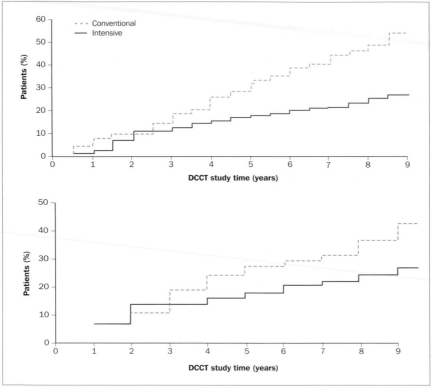

Figure 8. Comparison of conventional and intensive therapy in cumulative incidence of retinopathy progression (**top**) and microalbuminuria (**bottom**). Reproduced with permission from the American Medical Association.

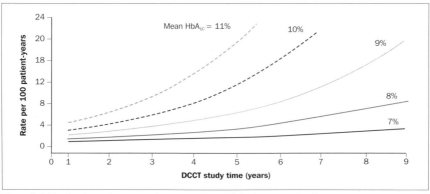

Figure 9. Risk of retinopathy progression versus mean HbA$_{1c}$ in conventional treatment group. Reproduced with permission from the American Medical Association.

Commentary

The value of intensive treatment of type 1 diabetes in preventing/slowing the development of microvascular disease was established by the DCCT. This study reported further follow-up of the same cohort of patients. It clearly shows that an earlier, prolonged period of intensive insulin treatment is associated with a reduced risk of microvascular complications compared with conventional treatment. The absolute risks of retinopathy and nephropathy were proportional to mean HbA_{1c} and, importantly, the benefits of intensive treatment extended well beyond the period of intensification.

This emphasises the point that early aggressive treatment of type 1 diabetes is vital to achieve good long-term diabetic control, and that the effects of this persist for many years. What the trial does not tell us is whether such intensification will produce similar benefits once complications have become established, or even reverse the problem.

The DCCT programme has described a clear path to establishing targets for diabetes control, and helped in the development of methodologies to achieve this.

Cardiovascular Mortality

Diabetes, plasma insulin and cardiovascular disease. Subgroup analysis from the Department of Veterans Affairs High-Density Lipoprotein Intervention Trial (VA-HIT)

What does this trial tell us?

➤ In men with coronary heart disease and low high-density lipoprotein (HDL) cholesterol, gemfibrozil reduces the risk of cardiovascular events in:

1. diabetic patients

2. non-diabetic patients with high fasting plasma insulin

Authors	Rubins HB, Robins SJ, Collins D, et al, for the VA-HIT Study Group
Reference	*Arch Intern Med* 2002;162:2597–604
Objectives	1. To determine the efficacy of gemfibrozil in patients with varying levels of glucose tolerance or hyperinsulinaemia
	2. To examine the association between diabetes status and glucose and insulin levels and risk of cardiovascular outcomes
Methodology	Subgroup analysis from the Department of Veterans Affairs High-Density Lipoprotein Intervention Trial, comparing gemfibrozil with placebo (*N Engl J Med* 1999;341:410–18)
Drugs used	Gemfibrozil 1,200 mg/day
Patients	2,531 men with coronary heart disease, HDL cholesterol ≤1.04 mmol/L and low-density lipoprotein cholesterol ≤3.63 mmol/L
Outcomes	Composite endpoint of coronary heart disease death, stroke or myocardial infarction
Analysis	Intention to treat. Risks compared with Cox proportional hazard models
Follow-up	Average 5.1 years

Results

Risk of cardiovascular composite endpoint				
	Diabetes*	Newly diagnosed diabetes*	Impaired fasting glucose (IFG)	Normal
Placebo group, %	36.5	34.3	23.8	21.0
Risk reduction in gemfibrozil group, %	32 (P=0.004)		18 (P=0.07) Highest quartile of IFG group: 25 (P=0.04)	
*Diabetic group versus non-diabetic group: P<0.001				

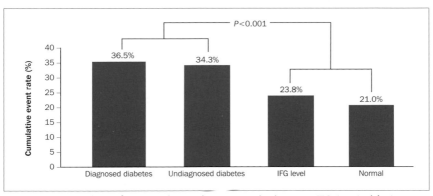

Figure 10. 5-year incidence of major cardiovascular events in placebo group. IFG: impaired fasting glucose. Reproduced with permission from the American Medical Association.

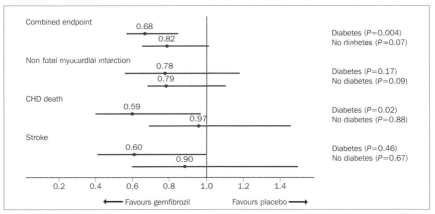

Figure 11. Hazard ratios for major cardiovascular events with gemfibrozil compared with placebo in subjects with and without diabetes. CHD: coronary heart disease. Reproduced with permission from the American Medical Association.

Commentary

It has long been known that high plasma insulin levels in non-diabetic subjects are associated with increased cardiovascular risk, and that this might be a reflection of insulin resistance and the metabolic syndrome. Similarly, diabetic subjects are at very high cardiovascular risk, and the typical dyslipidaemia of type 2 diabetes is low HDL cholesterol and raised triglycerides.

In this study, the effect of gemfibrozil, a fibrate agent that increases HDL cholesterol and lowers triglycerides, was studied as a subgroup analysis from the Department of Veterans Affairs High-Density Lipoprotein Intervention Trial. The aim was to determine the efficacy of gemfibrozil in subjects with varying levels of glucose intolerance or hyperinsulinaemia. The principal finding was that in men with coronary heart disease and low HDL cholesterol, gemfibrozil was associated with a reduced risk of cardiovascular events, both in diabetic and non-diabetic subjects with high fasting plasma insulin.

From the view of cardiovascular protection, the data are not currently as strong for fibrates as compared with statin agents. Further studies are ongoing in this area and will report in the next few years.

Effects of ramipril on cardiovascular and microvascular outcomes in people with diabetes mellitus: results of the HOPE study and MICRO-HOPE substudy

What does this trial tell us?

➤ The angiotensin-converting enzyme (ACE) inhibitor ramipril is beneficial for cardiovascular events and overt neuropathy in patients with diabetes

➤ The cardiovascular benefit is greater than that attributable to a decrease in blood pressure

➤ The treatment represents a vasculoprotective and renoprotective effect for patients with diabetes

Authors	Heart Outcomes Prevention Evaluation (HOPE) Study Investigators
Reference	*Lancet* 2000;355:253–9
Objective	To investigate whether ramipril can lower the risk of cardiovascular and renal disease in diabetes
Methodology	Two-by-two factorial design with randomisation of patients to ramipril or placebo
Drugs used	Ramipril 10 mg/day; vitamin E 400 IU/day (all patients)
Patients	3,577 patients with diabetes, aged ≥55 years, with a previous cardiovascular event or at least one other cardiovascular risk factor, with no proteinuria, heart failure or low ejection fraction at baseline, and who were not taking ACE inhibitors
Outcomes	The combined primary endpoint was myocardial infarction, stroke or cardiovascular death. Overt nephropathy was the primary endpoint in a substudy
Analysis	Intention to treat
Follow-up	4.5 years (study stopped 6 months early because of a consistent benefit of ramipril)

Results

Outcome	Ramipril, n (%)	Placebo, n (%)	% Relative risk reduction	P value
Primary outcome				
Combined	277 (15.3)	351 (19.8)	25	0.0004
Myocardial infarction	185 (10.2)	229 (12.9)	22	0.01
Stroke	76 (4.2)	108 (6.1)	33	0.0074
Cardiovascular death	112 (6.2)	172 (9.7)	37	0.0001
Secondary and other outcomes				
Total mortality	196 (10.8)	248 (14.0)	24	0.004
Revascularisation	254 (14.0)	291 (16.4)	17	0.031
Overt nephropathy	273 (15.1)	312 (17.6)	16	0.036

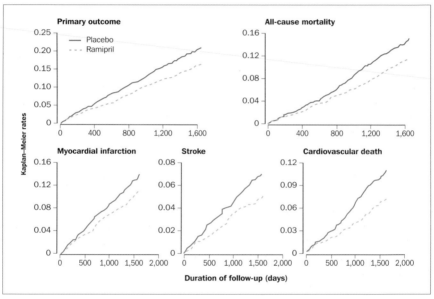

Figure 12. Kaplan–Meier survival curves for diabetic patients treated with ramipril or placebo. Reproduced with permission from *The Lancet*.

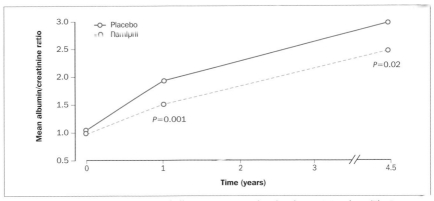

Figure 13. Effect of ramipril on degree of albuminuria. Reproduced with permission from *The Lancet*.

Commentary

This oft-quoted study investigated whether the ACE inhibitor ramipril is associated with a reduced risk of cardiovascular and renal disease in diabetes. This was part of a much larger study in high-risk patients. Around 3,500 patients with diabetes and a previous cardiovascular event or at least one cardiovascular risk factor were randomised to receive either ramipril 10 mg/day or placebo. Subjects in both the active and control groups could receive appropriate cardioprotective drugs and attained similar blood pressures. The use of ramipril was associated with a significant reduction in the combined primary endpoint.

The results of both HOPE and the Micro-HOPE substudy have been claimed by the authors to suggest a cardioprotective benefit with the use of ACE inhibitors, over and above that of blood pressure lowering alone. This explanation has been challenged, since there were small differences in blood pressure in favour of the ramipril group. Further work in this area is ongoing. In the meantime, inhibitors of the renin–angiotensin system are an important part of the armamentarium of drugs to treat hypertension in type 2 diabetic patients, and are also extremely useful in patients with heart failure. They should certainly be routinely used in diabetic patients with hypertension.

Mortality from coronary heart disease in subjects with type 2 diabetes and in non-diabetic subjects with and without prior myocardial infarction

What does this trial tell us?

➤ Diabetic patients without a previous myocardial infarction (MI) have as high a risk of MI as non-diabetic patients with a previous MI

➤ These data provide a rationale for aggressive treatment of cardiovascular risk factors in diabetic patients

Authors	Haffner SM, Lehto S, Rönnemaa T, et al
Reference	*N Engl J Med* 1998;339:229–34
Objective	To compare the risk of MI in diabetic patients who have not had an MI with the risk in non-diabetic patients who have had an MI
Methodology	Analysis of 7-year incidence rates of MI in diabetic and non-diabetic subjects with and without previous MI, adjusted for age, sex and major risk factors
Patients	1,059 patients with type 2 diabetes and 1,378 non-diabetic subjects, aged 45–64 years
Outcomes	7-year incidence of MI, 7-year risk of death from coronary heart disease
Analysis	Group differences assessed by logistic regression; Kaplan–Meier survival curves used to construct figures for mortality from coronary heart disease
Follow-up	7 years

Results

Outcome	Non-diabetic subjects		Diabetic subjects	
	Prior MI	No prior MI	Prior MI	No Prior MI
7-year incidence rate of MI	18.8%	3.5% (P<0.001)	45.0%	20.2% (P<0.001)

The hazard ratio for death from coronary heart disease for diabetic subjects without prior MI compared with non-diabetic subjects with MI was not significantly different from 1.0

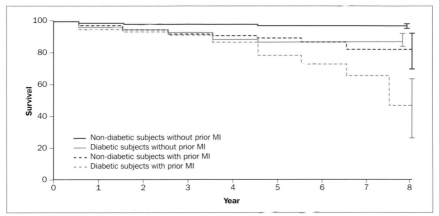

Figure 14. Kaplan–Meier estimates of probabilities of death from coronary heart disease in diabetic and non-diabetic subjects, with and without prior myocardial infarction (MI). Reproduced with permission from the Massachusetts Medical Society.

Commentary

This oft-quoted paper helped to emphasise that type 2 diabetes is a cardiovascular disease. Diabetic patients *without* a history of prior MI were at just as high risk of having an MI as non-diabetic patients *with* a history of prior MI. This paper suggests that the concept of primary prevention in diabetes is dead – all patients with diabetes, whether they have had a prior cardiovascular event or not, should be treated from a secondary preventative point of view. This study, and others published more recently looking at cardiovascular risk intervention, implies that all type 2 diabetic patients should be prescribed cardioprotective drugs, particularly statins, unless there is a contraindication or tolerability problem.

Glucose tolerance and mortality: comparison of WHO and American Diabetic Association diagnostic criteria

What does this trial tell us?

➤ Fasting glucose concentrations alone do not identify patients at increased risk of death associated with hyperglycaemia

➤ The oral glucose tolerance test provides additional prognostic information and enables the detection of patients with impaired glucose tolerance, who have the greatest risk of death

Authors	Diabetes Epidemiology: Collaborative Analysis of Diagnostic Criteria in Europe (DECODE) Study Group for the European Diabetes Epidemiology Group
Reference	*Lancet* 1999;354:617–21
Objective	To assess mortality associated with the American Diabetic Association (ADA) fasting glucose criteria (newly diagnosed diabetes: ≥7.0 mmol/L; impaired fasting glucose: 6.1–6.9 mmol/L) compared with the World Health Organization (WHO) 2-hour post-challenge glucose criteria (newly diagnosed diabetes: ≥11.1 mmol/L; impaired fasting glucose: 7.8–11.1 mmol/L)
Methodology	Assessment of baseline data on glucose concentrations at fasting and 2 hours after a 75 g oral glucose tolerance test from 13 prospective European cohort studies
Patients	18,048 men and 7,316 women aged ≥30 years, 1,275 previously diagnosed with diabetes
Outcome	All-cause mortality
Analysis	Mortality for various glucose categories calculated using Cox's proportional hazards model
Follow-up	Mean 7.3 years

Results

Hazard ratios for death (compared with individuals with normal fasting glucose)				
Glucose criteria	Newly diagnosed diabetes		Impaired fasting glucose (7.8–11.1 mmol/L)	
	Men	Women	Men	Women
ADA	1.81	1.79	1.21	1.08
WHO	2.02	2.77	1.51	1.60

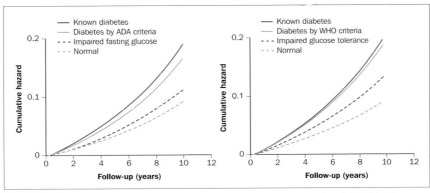

Figure 15. Cumulative hazard curves for (**left**) ADA fasting glucose criteria and (**right**) WHO 2-hour glucose criteria adjusted for age, sex and study centre. Reproduced with permission from *The Lancet.*

Commentary

There has been longstanding controversy about the relative merits of different screening tests and reference ranges for the diagnosis of diabetes and impaired glucose tolerance. Moreover, it has been well reported that both impaired glucose tolerance and type 2 diabetes are associated with significantly increased cardiovascular risk. It is particularly important, then, that any screening tests for abnormalities of glycaemia accurately reflect that risk.

In this study, a comparison was made of the ADA and WHO diagnostic criteria for glucose dysregulation. The objective was to assess mortality using fasting glucose and 2-hour post-challenge glucose values (75 g oral glucose tolerance test), respectively. The principal finding was that the 2-hour post-challenge glucose value was more predictive of all-cause mortality than the fasting glucose value. The researchers found that the oral glucose tolerance test remains a useful investigation in providing additional prognostic information and, in particular, allows the detection of patients with impaired glucose tolerance who have the greatest risk of death.

Lipids

Effect of fenofibrate on progression of coronary-artery disease in type 2 diabetes: the Diabetes Atherosclerosis Intervention Study, a randomised study

What does this trial tell us?

➤ Treatment with fenofibrate reduces the progression of coronary artery disease in type 2 diabetes

➤ The effect is at least partly related to correction of lipoprotein abnormalities, even in patients not previously judged to need lipid-lowering treatment

Authors	Diabetes Atherosclerosis Intervention Study Investigators
Reference	*Lancet* 2001;357:905–10
Objective	To assess the effects of correcting lipoprotein abnormalities on coronary atherosclerosis in type 2 diabetes
Methodology	Randomised controlled trial of fenofibrate versus placebo
Drugs used	Fenofibrate 200 mg/day
Patients	418 patients with type 2 diabetes with good glycaemic control, mild lipoprotein abnormalities and at least one coronary lesion visible on angiography: 201 randomised to fenofibrate (mean age 57 years), 211 randomised to placebo (mean age 56 years)
Outcomes	Plasma cholesterol, high-density lipoprotein (HDL) and low-density lipoprotein (LDL) cholesterol and triglyceride levels; coronary artery stenosis diameter, lumen diameter, mean segment diameter
Analysis	Intention to treat
Follow-up	At least 3 years

Results

Outcome	Comment
Lipid concentrations	Total plasma cholesterol, HDL and LDL cholesterol and triglyceride levels all changed significantly more in the fenofibrate group than in the placebo group ($P<0.001$, see **Figure 16**)

Outcome	Placebo	Fenofibrate	P value
Coronary artery disease			
Increase in percentage diameter stenosis	3.65	2.11	0.02
Decrease in minimum lumen diameter	−0.10	−0.06	0.029
Decrease in mean segment diameter	−0.08	−0.06	0.171

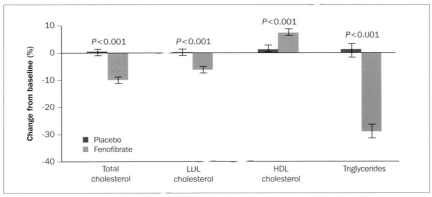

Figure 16. Changes in lipid values in placebo and fenofibrate groups. HDL: high-density lipoprotein; LDL: low-density lipoprotein. Reproduced with permission from *The Lancet*.

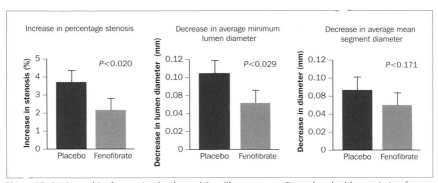

Figure 17. Angiographic changes in placebo and fenofibrate groups. Reproduced with permission from *The Lancet*.

37

Commentary

Although statins remain the mainstay of treatment for dyslipidaemia in those with high cardiovascular risk, these agents are more specific in targeting LDL cholesterol and do little for HDL cholesterol or triglycerides. Fibrates, however, are peroxisome proliferator-activated receptor alpha agonists that act to raise HDL and lower triglycerides.

Given that low HDL and raised triglycerides are commonly found in type 2 diabetes and the metabolic syndrome, this was a logical study to determine whether fenofibrate would reduce the progression of coronary artery disease in type 2 diabetes. The study was positive based on an improvement in surrogate markers of progression of coronary artery disease. The findings are insufficient to recommend blanket treatment of type 2 diabetics with fibrate agents, but further hard endpoint studies are awaited. These will hopefully determine the place of fibrate agents in clinical practice.

Reduced coronary events in simvastatin-treated patients with coronary heart disease and diabetes or impaired fasting glucose levels. Subgroup analyses in the Scandinavian Simvastatin Survival Study

What does this trial tell us?

➤ Simvastatin-treated diabetic patients have a significantly reduced risk of major coronary events and revascularisations

➤ Simvastatin-treated patients with impaired fasting glucose have a significantly reduced risk of major coronary events, revascularisations and total and coronary mortality

Authors	Haffner SM, Alexander CM, Cook TJ, et al, for the Scandinavian Simvastatin Survival Study Group
Reference	*Arch Intern Med* 1999;159:2661–7
Objective	To examine the effect of simvastatin therapy on coronary heart disease (CHD) in patients with diabetes and impaired fasting glucose levels
Methodology	Subgroup analysis of a double-blind, randomised, placebo-controlled multicentre trial of long-term simvastatin therapy in patients with CHD (*Diabetes Care* 1997;20:614–20)
Drugs used	Simvastatin, dose titrated to a serum cholesterol level of 3.0–5.2 mmol/L
Patients	3,237 patients with normal fasting glucose, 678 with impaired fasting glucose and 483 with diabetes
Outcomes	The primary endpoint was total mortality. Secondary endpoints were major coronary events and non-fatal myocardial infarction. Tertiary endpoints included any CHD event and revascularisation
Analysis	Effect of simvastatin treatment was assessed by calculating relative risk with the Cox regression model
Follow-up	Average 5.4 years

Results

Major coronary events	Normal fasting glucose	Impaired fasting glucose	Diabetes
Simvastatin group, n (%)	299 (18.6)	67 (19.5)	59 (23.5)
Placebo group, n (%)	428 (26.2)	102 (30.5)	87 (37.5)
Relative risk	0.68	0.624	0.581
P for relative risk	<0.001	0.003	0.001

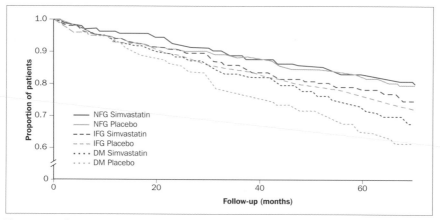

Figure 18. Kaplan–Meier survival curves for the probability of remaining free of a major coronary heart disease event during follow-up in placebo- and simvastatin-treated patients with normal fasting glucose (NFG), impaired fasting glucose (IFG) and diabetes mellitus (DM). Reproduced with permission from the American Medical Association.

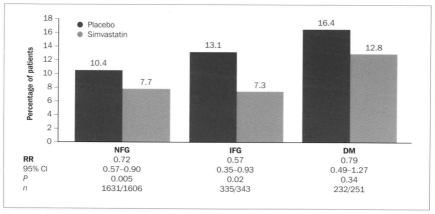

Figure 19. Incidence of total mortality and relative risk (RR) by glucose status in patients treated with simvastatin and placebo. CI: confidence interval; DM: diabetes mellitus; IFG: impaired fasting glucose; NFG: normal fasting glucose. Reproduced with permission from the American Medical Association.

Commentary

This was a subgroup analysis of the Scandinavian Simvastatin Survival Study (4S). 4S had already demonstrated a profound benefit in reducing cardiovascular events and mortality by using statin agents in secondary prevention. Subgroup analysis in the diabetic cohort demonstrated a significantly reduced risk of major coronary events and revascularisations. This was also true of patients with impaired glucose tolerance.

This was one of the first hard endpoint clinical trials of statins, which are now widely used for both primary and secondary prevention of cardiovascular disease. More recent studies have supported the proposition that all type 2 diabetic patients should be on a statin agent unless there is a contraindication or tolerability problem.

The cost-effectiveness of lipid lowering in patients with diabetes: results from the 4S trial

What does this trial tell us?

➤ For patients with diabetes, treatment with simvastatin results in estimates of cost per life-year gained that are well within the range generally considered cost-effective

➤ Simvastatin therapy appears to provide good value for money in both diabetic and non-diabetic patients with cardiovascular disease

Authors	Jönsson B, Cook JR, Pedersen TR
Reference	*Diabetologia* 1999;42:1293–301
Objective	To investigate the cost-effectiveness of simvastatin in patients with diabetes
Methodology	Randomised controlled trial comparing simvastatin with placebo
Drugs used	Simvastatin 20–40 mg; insulin and oral hypoglycaemic drugs as indicated by fasting blood glucose
Patients	4,444 patients, aged 35–70 years, from five Nordic countries, with prior myocardial infarction, angina or both
Outcomes	Cost-effectiveness related to life-years gained from reduction in mortality
Analysis	Intention to treat. Cost-effectiveness ratios estimated as ratio of incremental cost of intervention to the gain in life-years for patients randomised to simvastatin compared with placebo
Follow-up	Mean 5.5 years

Results

	Hospital costs (Swedish Kroners)			Prescription costs		Total costs	
	Simvastatin	Placebo	Difference	Simvastatin	% Offset	Simvastatin	Placebo
Non-diabetic	16,899	24,631	−7,732	22,195	34.8	39,093	24,631
Diabetic	21,730	35,943	−14,213	21,246	66.9	42,975	35,943

Cost per life-year gained ranged from €1,554 for diabetic patients to €7,345 for patients with normal fasting glucose. Data from the other Nordic countries (Denmark, Finland, Iceland and Norway) were comparable

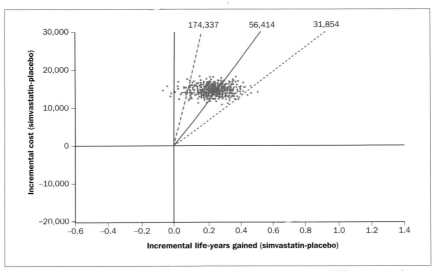

Figure 20. Scatterplot of 1,000 bootstrap replicates showing incremental cost and life-years gained in non-diabetic subjects. The solid line represents the cost-effectiveness ratio (incremental cost per life-year gained) estimate. The dashed lines show the 95% bootstrap confidence intervals. Costs are in Swedish Kroners. Reproduced with permission from Springer-Verlag.

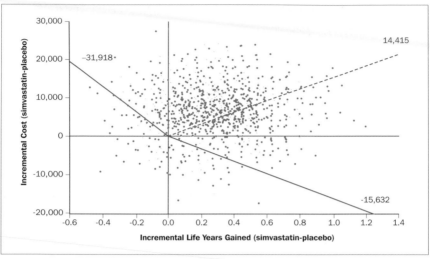

Figure 21. Scatterplot of 1,000 bootstrap replicates showing incremental cost and life-years gained in diabetic patients. The solid line represents the cost-effectiveness ratio (incremental cost per life-year gained) estimate. The dashed lines show the 95% bootstrap confidence intervals. Costs are in Swedish Kroners. Reproduced with permission from Springer-Verlag.

Commentary

This was a further study to arise from the 4S trial. This trial looked at the cost-effectiveness of simvastatin in patients with diabetes. Cost per life-year gained for diabetic patients was around £1,000 (€1,554), ie, extremely cost-effective. It is this type of study that has laid to rest the idea that our health service cannot afford statin treatment. It is one of the most cost-effective treatments we have, giving significant reductions in morbidity and mortality, principally from cardiovascular events in higher-risk patients, including those with diabetes.

Effect of niacin on lipid and lipoprotein levels and glycemic control in patients with diabetes and peripheral arterial disease. The ADMIT study: a randomised trial

What does this trial tell us?

➤ Lipid-modifying doses of niacin can be safely used in patients with diabetes

➤ Niacin therapy can be an effective alternative where statins or fibrates are not tolerated or where they fail to correct hypertriglyceridaemia or low high density lipoprotein (HDL) cholesterol levels

Authors	Elam MB, Hunninghake DB, Davis BK, et al, for the Arterial Disease Multiple Intervention Trial (ADMIT) Investigators
Reference	*JAMA* 2000;284:1263–70
Objective	To determine the efficacy and safety of lipid-modifying doses of niacin in patients with diabetes
Methodology	Prospective, randomised, six-centre controlled study of niacin versus placebo, following an active niacin run-in
Drugs used	Niacin 3,000 mg/day or maximum tolerated dose
Patients	468 patients with peripheral arterial disease, including 125 with diabetes
Outcomes	Main outcome measures included levels of plasma lipoproteins and HbA_{1c}, hypoglycaemic drug use, compliance and adverse events
Analysis	Effects of niacin treatment and safety parameters, each analysed with a longitudinal regression model
Follow-up	60 weeks

45

Results

Effect of niacin on lipid and lipoprotein levels from baseline to week 18

	Baseline	Week 18	% Change
Cholesterol (mg/dL)			
Placebo	217	220	1.4
Niacin	207	198	−4.3*
Triglycerides (mg/dL)			
Placebo	197	210	6.6
Niacin	176	136	−22.7*
HDL cholesterol (mg/dL)			
Placebo	39	39	0
Niacin	38	49	28.9*
LDL cholesterol (mg/dL)			
Placebo	138	139	0.7
Niacin	133	122	−8.3*

*$P < 0.001$ versus placebo

Effect of niacin on average plasma glucose in patients with and without diabetes

	With diabetes				Without diabetes			
	Baseline	Week 18	% Change	P value	Baseline	Week 18	% Change	P value
Glucose (mg/dL)								
Placebo	165	157	−8.7		96	97	0.5	
Niacin	165	173	8.1	0.04	95	102	6.3	≤ 0.001

There was no evidence of sustained niacin-induced impairment of glycaemic control

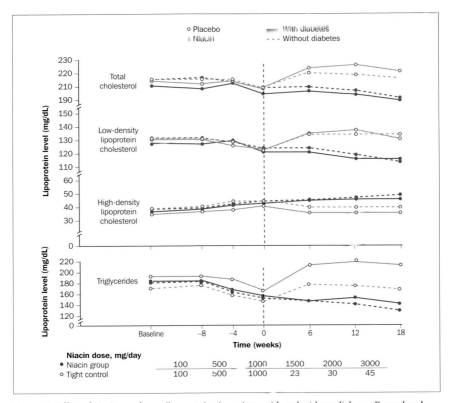

Figure 22. Effect of niacin on plasma lipoproteins in patients with and without diabetes. Reproduced with permission from the American Medical Association.

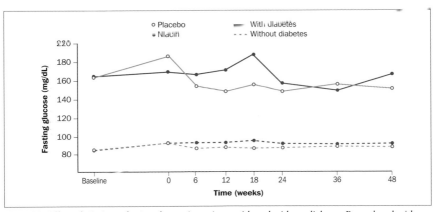

Figure 23. Effect of niacin on fasting glucose in patients with and without diabetes. Reproduced with permission from the American Medical Association.

Commentary

Although statin agents have unequivocally been shown to reduce the risks of cardiovascular events in higher-risk subjects, it is clear that this reduction is not absolute. People with diabetes commonly have a range of lipid abnormalities, particularly low HDL cholesterol and raised triglycerides. In this study, niacin (a nicotinic acid derivative that has been shown to lower triglycerides and increase HDL cholesterol) was studied to determine its efficacy and safety in patients with diabetes. The authors found that lipid-modifying doses of niacin can be safely used in diabetic patients, and that niacin might be an alternative to statins or fibrates if these are not tolerated or where the lipid abnormalities warrant its use.

Although this was not a landmark study, it laid the ground for other (ongoing) studies. These are looking at the endpoint effects of agents that not only lower LDL cholesterol (ie, statins), but also have positive effects on other lipid abnormalities, such as HDL cholesterol and triglycerides.

Importantly, this study found no evidence of further impairment of glucose intolerance in diabetic patients with niacin, as had been suggested in previous commentaries on this agent.

MRC/BHF Heart Protection Study of cholesterol-lowering with simvastatin in 5,963 people with diabetes: a randomised placebo-controlled trial

What does this trial tell us?

➤ Cholesterol-lowering therapy is beneficial for patients with diabetes, even if they do not already have manifest coronary heart disease or a high cholesterol concentration

➤ Statin therapy should be considered routinely for diabetic patients at elevated risk of major vascular events, irrespective of initial cholesterol concentrations

Authors	Heart Protection Study Collaborative Group
Reference	*Lancet* 2003;361:2005–16
Objective	To investigate the effects of lowering cholesterol in patients with diabetes
Methodology	Randomised controlled trial of simvastatin versus matching placebo
Drugs used	Simvastatin 40 mg/day
Patients	5,963 patients, aged 40–80 years, with diabetes, and 14,573 with occlusive arterial disease but no diabetes
Outcomes	Primary endpoints were first major coronary event (eg, non-fatal myocardial infarction or coronary death) and first major vascular event (eg, stroke, revascularisation). Secondary endpoints included subsequent vascular events
Analysis	Main comparisons involved log-rank analysis of the first occurrence of specific events following randomisation (intention to treat)
Follow-up	Means of 4.8 years for patients with diabetes at study entry and 5.0 years for all other participants

Results

Effects of simvastatin allocation on first major coronary event, stroke or revascularisation				
Major vascular event and prior disease group	Simvastatin-allocated, n (%)	Placebo-allocated, n (%)	Event ratio	P value
Major coronary event				
Diabetes	279 (9.4)	377 (12.6)		
No diabetes	619 (8.5)	835 (11.5)		
Subtotal	898 (8.7)	1,212 (11.8)	0.73	<0.0001
Stroke				
Diabetes	149 (5.0)	193 (6.5)		
No diabetes	295 (4.0)	392 (5.4)		
Subtotal	444 (4.3)	585 (5.7)	0.75	<0.0001
Revascularisation				
Diabetes	260 (8.7)	309 (10.4)		
No diabetes	679 (9.3)	896 (12.3)		
Subtotal	939 (9.1)	1,205 (11.7)	0.76	<0.0001
Major vascular event				
Diabetes	601 (20.2)	748 (25.1)		
No diabetes	1,432 (19.6)	1,837 (25.2)		
Subtotal	2,033 (19.8)	2,585 (25.2)	0.76	<0.0001

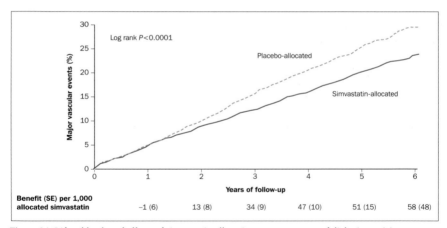

Figure 24. Life-table plot of effects of simvastatin allocation on percentages of diabetic participants having major vascular events. SE: standard error. Reproduced with permission from *The Lancet*.

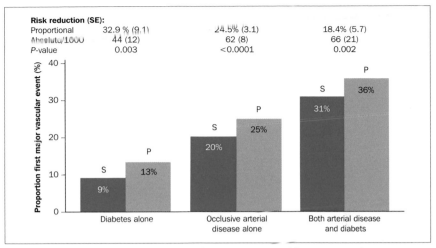

Figure 25. Absolute effects of simvastatin allocation on 5-year rates of first major vascular event. P: placebo-allocated; S: simvastatin-allocated; SE: standard error. Reproduced with permission from *The Lancet.*

Commentary

This landmark trial investigated the effects of lowering total and low-density lipoprotein cholesterol in a large group of patients (almost 6,000 with diabetes). The study was a randomised controlled trial of simvastatin 40 mg/day versus placebo. There were clear and profound risk reductions in the active treatment group both for diabetic and non-diabetic patients.

Given that type 2 diabetes is a cardiovascular disease and this latter kills the vast majority of patients, it is now hard to argue with the concept that all type 2 diabetic patients should be on a statin agent unless there is a contraindication or tolerability problem (see also CARDS, p. 52).

Primary prevention of cardiovascular disease with atorvastatin in type 2 diabetes in the Collaborative Atorvastatin Diabetes Study (CARDS): multicentre randomised placebo-controlled trial

What does this trial tell us?

➤ Atorvastatin 10 mg/day is safe and efficacious in reducing the risk of first cardiovascular events in patients with type 2 diabetes, without high low-density lipoprotein (LDL) cholesterol

➤ There appears to be no justification for having a particular LDL cholesterol threshold at which patients with type 2 diabetes should have statins

Authors	Colhoun HM, Betteridge DJ, Durrington PN, et al, for the CARDS Investigators
Reference	*Lancet* 2004;364:685–96
Objective	To assess the effectiveness of atorvastatin for the primary prevention of major cardiovascular events in patients with type 2 diabetes and without high LDL cholesterol
Methodology	Randomised controlled study of atorvastatin versus placebo
Drugs used	Atorvastatin 10 mg/day
Patients	2,838 patients, aged 40–75 years, with no history of cardiovascular disease, LDL cholesterol ≤4.14 mmol/L, fasting triglyceride ≤6.78 mmol/L and at least one of retinopathy, albuminuria, current smoking or hypertension
Outcomes	The primary endpoint was time to first occurrence of one of an acute coronary heart disease event, coronary revascularisation or stroke. Secondary endpoints included death from any cause and any acute cardiovascular event
Analysis	Intention to treat
Follow-up	Median 3.9 years

Results

Number of patients with an event (%)				
Outcome	Placebo	Atorvastatin 10 mg	Hazard ratio	P value
Primary endpoint	127 (9.0)	83 (5.8)	0.63	0.001
Acute coronary events	77 (5.5)	51 (3.6)	0.64	
Coronary revascularisation	34 (2.4)	24 (1.7)	0.69	
Stroke	39 (2.8)	21 (1.5)	0.52	
Secondary endpoint				
Death from any cause	82 (5.8)	61 (4.3)	0.73	0.059
Any acute cardiovascular event	189 (13.4)	134 (9.4)	0.68	0.001

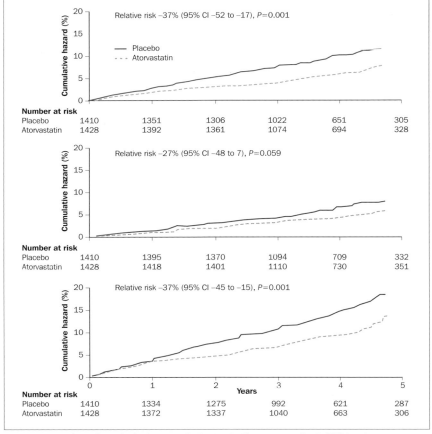

Figure 26. Cumulative hazard of primary endpoint (**top**), all-cause mortality (**middle**) and any cardiovascular endpoint (**bottom**). CI: confidence interval. Reproduced with permission from *The Lancet*.

Commentary

This landmark lipid study specifically randomised a large group of patients with type 2 diabetes who did not have particularly high LDL cholesterol to receive either atorvastatin 10 mg/day or placebo. During follow-up there were significant risk reductions in both the primary and secondary endpoints. Atorvastatin was found to be safe and efficacious, and the trial was stopped early because the results were so impressive.

This study supports the earlier Heart Protection Study (see p. 49), which showed the same level of benefit (from the point of view of reduction of cardiovascular events) at every level of starting cholesterol in high-risk subjects. Therefore, there appears to be no justification for advising statin usage only above a certain level of LDL cholesterol – all type 2 diabetic patients benefit from statin usage, whatever their level of cholesterol. Since they are at such high risk of cardiovascular disease, all type 2 diabetic patients should be treated with a statin – ie, the concept of primary prevention in type 2 diabetes is redundant.

Cost-Effectiveness

Implementing intensive control of blood glucose concentration and blood pressure in type 2 diabetes in England: cost analysis (UKPDS 63)

What does this trial tell us?

➤ Policies to improve control of blood glucose and blood pressure in type 2 diabetes are effective in reducing complications, and are also cost-effective

➤ The total cost represents only a small fraction of National Health Service (NHS) spending plans

Authors	Gray A, Clarke P, Farmer A, Holman R, for the UK Prospective Diabetes Study (UKPDS) Group
Reference	*BMJ* 2002;325:860
Objective	To estimate the incremental cost of implementing policies for intensive control of blood glucose concentration and blood pressure for all patients with type 2 diabetes in England
Methodology	Extrapolation of resource use and cost data derived from a randomised controlled trial (*Lancet* 1998;352:837–53)
Drugs used	Hypoglycaemic and antihypertensive drugs as required to maintain intensive control of blood glucose (tighter than conventional control, defined as plasma glucose concentration <15 mmol/L) and of blood pressure (tighter than conventional control, defined as blood pressure <180/105 mm Hg)
Patients	Trial population (5,102 patients with newly diagnosed type 2 diabetes) extrapolated to the total population of England with type 2 diabetes (calculated as 2.5% of the population aged ≥16 years, or 1.011 million individuals)
Outcomes	Total costs based on use of healthcare resources, including costs of management, treatment and hospitalisation
Analysis	Sensitivity analysis performed on key variables subject to uncertainty; all results reported in pounds sterling at 1999 prices

Results

Estimated total cost of adopting policies for intensive control of blood glucose and blood pressure control in England (1999 £). Values are £m unless otherwise stated				
Age group (years)	Management	Treatment	Complications	Total
<45	16.8	7.4	-3.9	20.3
45–49	8.9	4.3	-2.4	10.9
50–54	9.6	4.7	-3.6	10.7
55–59	14.8	7.6	-8.0	14.3
60–64	13.1	7.1	-10.5	9.7
65–70	18.1	10.4	-17.6	10.9
>70	50.6	31.3	-58.2	23.7
Total	132.0	72.8	-104.2	100.5
Total per person treated (£)	193	107	-153	147

Net annual cost of intensive blood glucose and blood pressure control in all patients with type 2 diabetes in England is estimated at £100.5m ($156m, €159m), which is less than 1% of the proposed annual NHS expenditure in 2001–5

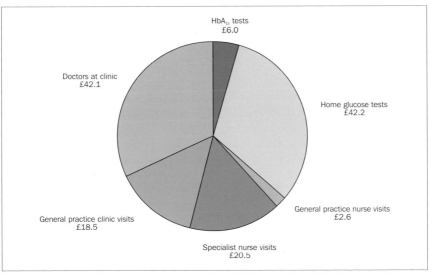

Figure 27. Estimated additional management costs (£m, 1999) of adopting policies in England for intensive control of blood glucose and blood pressure (total=£132m). Reproduced with permission from BMJ Publishing.

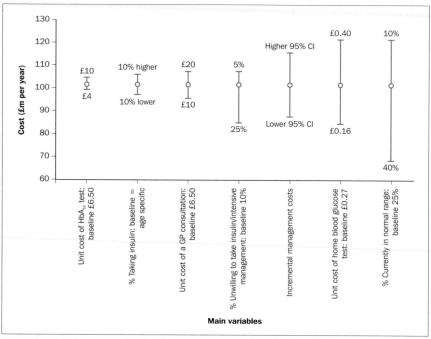

Figure 28. Sensitivity analysis showing the impact on estimated total cost of changes in the main variables (baseline total=£100.5m). CI: confidence interval. Reproduced with permission from BMJ Publishing.

Commentary

In this further study from the UKPDS Group, the authors attempted to estimate the incremental cost of implementing policies for intensive control of blood glucose and blood pressure for all patients with type 2 diabetes in England. They based their findings on UKPDS data, and concluded that policies to improve control of blood glucose and blood pressure in type 2 diabetes are cost-effective and would reduce the risk of long-term complications. They pointed out that the total cost is only a small fraction of the NHS spending generally and on diabetes in particular. The majority of costs relating to diabetes treatment (around 80%) relate to the long-term complications of this disease; effective prevention is therefore very likely to be cost-effective.

Cost effectiveness of an intensive blood glucose control policy in patients with type 2 diabetes: economic analysis alongside randomised controlled trial (UKPDS 41)

What does this trial tell us?

➤ Intensive blood glucose control in type 2 diabetes significantly increases treatment costs, but substantially increases time free from complications and reduces the cost of complications

➤ In a UK primary care practice with 10,000 patients, additional costs would be £14,000–£27,000, but these would be offset by £10,000–£18,000 savings on complications

Authors	Gray A, Raikou M, McGuire A, et al, for the UK Prospective Diabetes Study (UKPDS) Group
Reference	*BMJ* 2000;320:1373–8
Objective	To estimate the cost-effectiveness of intensive versus conventional blood glucose control in type 2 diabetes
Methodology	Incremental cost-effectiveness analysis alongside a randomised controlled trial of intensive glucose control versus conventional management
Drugs used	Conventional management mainly through diet (aimed at fasting plasma glucose [FPG] <15 mmol/L); intensive management with insulin or sulphonylureas aimed at FPG <6 mmol/L
Patients	3,867 patients, mean age 53 years, with type 2 diabetes (defined as FPG >6 mmol/L) without symptoms of hyperglycaemia
Outcomes	The primary endpoint was incremental cost per event-free year gained within the trial period. Secondary endpoints included diabetes-related death and all-cause mortality
Analysis	Intention to treat
Follow-up	15 years

Results

Mean costs and effects for intensive and conventional blood glucose control policies			
Item	Intensive	Conventional	Mean difference
Mean cost/patient (1997 £)			
Routine treatment	4,350	3,655	695
Treatment of complications	5,258	6,215	−957
Mean event-free years/patient			
Within-trial event-free years	14.89	14.29	0.60
Estimated lifetime event-free years	15.08	13.94	1.14
Incremental cost per event-free year gained was £1,166 (costs and effects discounted at 6% per year)			

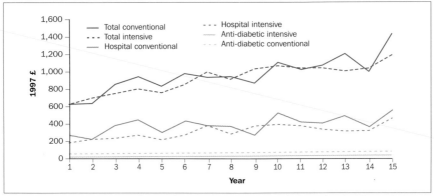

Figure 29. Mean cost per patient by year from randomisation (1997 £). Reproduced with permission from BMJ Publishing.

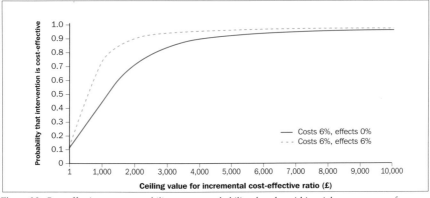

Figure 30. Cost-effectiveness acceptability curves: probability that the within-trial cost per event-free year gained is cost-effective (y axis) as a function of the decision maker's cost-effectiveness ratio (x axis). Reproduced with permission from BMJ Publishing.

Commentary

This study aimed to determine whether intensive blood glucose control in type 2 diabetes was cost-effective. The authors found that such an approach significantly increased treatment costs, but substantially increased time free from complications, thereby reducing the cost of such complications. Overall, intensive insulin treatment (leading to reduced risks of vascular complications) was found to be extremely cost-effective.

Nephropathy

Preventing microalbuminuria in type 2 diabetes

What does this trial tell us?

➤ Treatment with the angiotensin-converting enzyme (ACE) inhibitor trandolapril decreases the incidence of microalbuminuria in type 2 diabetes

➤ Addition of the non-dihydropyridine calcium-channel blocker verapamil does not appear to enhance the renoprotective effect of the ACE inhibitor

➤ The effect of verapamil alone is similar to that of placebo in this group of patients

Authors	Ruggenenti P, Fassi A, Ilieva AP, et al, for the Bergamo Nephrologic Diabetes Complications Trial (BENEDICT) Investigators
Reference	*N Engl J Med* 2004;351:1941–51
Objective	To assess whether ACE inhibitors and non-dihydropyridine calcium-channel blockers, alone or in combination, prevent microalbuminuria in patients with hypertension, type 2 diabetes and normal urinary albumin excretion
Methodology	Randomised controlled trial comparing the renoprotective effect of trandolapril plus verapamil, trandolapril alone, verapamil alone and placebo
Drugs used	Trandolapril 2 mg/day, verapamil 180 or 240 mg/day, additional antihypertensive drugs as necessary to achieve target blood pressure (≤120/80 mm Hg)
Patients	1,204 patients, aged ≥40 years, with hypertension and type 2 diabetes (diagnosed according to World Health Organization criteria)
Outcomes	The primary endpoint was development of persistent microalbuminuria. Secondary endpoints included blood pressure, serum creatinine, HbA_{1c} and cholesterol levels
Analysis	Analysis of the primary endpoint was with a survival analysis model
Follow-up	4 years

Results

Normal albumin excretion at baseline and during follow-up in patients receiving antihypertensive agents

Treatment	Baseline				Follow-up			
	Trandolapril, n (%)	Verapamil, n (%)	Verapamil + Trandolapril, n (%)	Placebo, n (%)	Trandolapril, n (%)	Verapamil, n (%)	Verapamil + Trandolapril n (%)	Placebo, n (%)
Any antihyper-tensive	172 (57.1)	162 (53.5)	161 (53.7)	169 (56.3)	193 (64.1)	188 (62.0)	165 * (55.0)	201 (67.0)
Diuretic	66 (21.9)	70 (23.1)	58 (19.3)	65 (21.7)	51 (16.9)	65 (21.5)	51 (17.0)	65 (21.7)
Beta-blocker	31 (10.3)	24 (7.9)	23 (7.7)	25 (8.3)	29 (9.6)	21 (6.9)	26 (8.7)	29 (9.7)
Calcium-channel blocker	73 (24.3)	88 (29.0)	87 (29.0)	90 (30.0)	79 (26.2)	77 * (25.4)	74 * (24.7)	98 (32.7)
Sympatholytic	68 (22.6)	63 (20.8)	59 (19.7)	56 (18.7)	137 * (45.5)	149 (49.2)	109 * (36.3)	163 (54.3)

*Significant difference compared with placebo

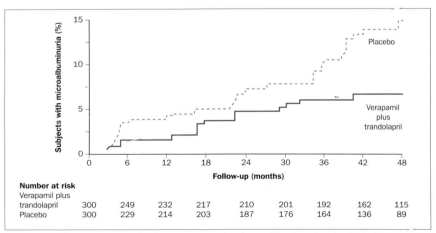

Number at risk

Verapamil plus trandolapril	300	249	232	217	210	201	192	162	115
Placebo	300	229	214	203	187	176	164	136	89

Figure 31. Kaplan–Meier curves for the percentages of patients with microalbuminuria during treatment with trandolapril plus verapamil or placebo. Reproduced with permission from the Massachusetts Medical Society.

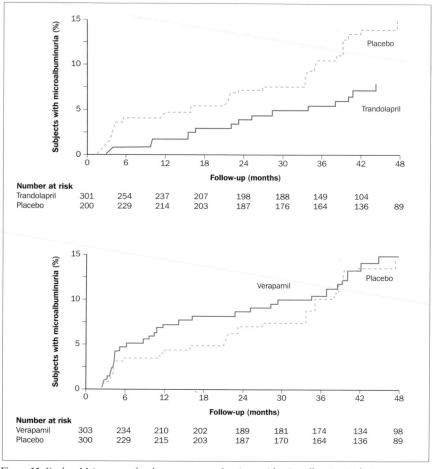

Figure 32. Kaplan–Meier curves for the percentages of patients with microalbuminuria during treatment with (top) trandolapril or placebo and (bottom) verapamil or placebo. Reproduced with permission from the Massachusetts Medical Society.

Commentary

This paper takes us back a stage further in examining the effects of inhibition of the renin–angiotensin system on the development of diabetic nephropathy.

Compared with placebo, treatment with an ACE inhibitor (trandolapril) or the combination of an ACE inhibitor and a calcium-channel blocker (verapamil) was associated with a significant risk reduction for the development of microalbuminuria over a 4-year period. Verapamil alone was not associated with such a protective effect.

This study emphasises the fact that blocking the renin–angiotensin system, specifically with ACE inhibition, is associated with renal protection (an effect not necessarily shown by other classes of antihypertensives). This study has profound implications for the use of ACE inhibitors (and presumably also angiotensin receptor blockers), even in type 2 diabetic patients with hypertension and no evidence of renal disease. The logical extension of the argument is that an inhibitor of the renin–angiotensin system should be a normal part of the pharmacotherapeutic armamentarium for all patients with type 2 diabetes and hypertension, irrespective of whether they yet have evidence of renal protein leakage.

Angiotensin-receptor blockade versus converting-enzyme inhibition in type 2 diabetes and nephropathy

What does this trial tell us?

➤ The angiotensin-II receptor blocker telmisartan is not inferior to the angiotensin-converting enzyme (ACE) inhibitor enalapril in providing long-term renoprotection in type 2 diabetes

➤ Results support the clinical equivalence of angiotensin-II receptor blockers and ACE inhibitors in patients at high risk for cardiovascular events

Authors	Barnett AH, Bain SC, Bouter P, et al, for the Diabetics Exposed to Telmisartan and Enalapril (DETAIL) Study Group
Reference	*N Engl J Med* 2004;351:1952–61
Objective	To compare the renoprotective effects of an angiotensin-II receptor blocker and an ACE inhibitor in type 2 diabetes
Methodology	Prospective, randomised, double-blind, double-dummy, parallel-group comparison of telmisartan and enalapril, conducted at 39 centres
Drugs used	Telmisartan 80 mg/day, enalapril 20 mg/day
Patients	250 adults with type 2 diabetes, mild to moderate hypertension and early nephropathy (based mainly on urinary albumin excretion rate and glomerular filtration rate)
Outcomes	The primary endpoint was change in glomerular filtration rate (determined by measuring plasma clearance of iohexol) between baseline and last available date. Secondary endpoints included: annual changes in glomerular filtration rate, serum creatinine level, urinary albumin excretion and blood pressure; rates of end-stage renal disease and cardiovascular events; rate of death from all causes
Analysis	Analysis of primary endpoint based on last observation carried forward
Follow-up	5 years

Results

Primary endpoint: changes in glomerular filtration rate per 1.73 m² (for a treatment difference of –3.0 mL per 1.73 m²)	
Telmisartan group (n=103)	–17.9 mL/minute
Enalapril group (n=113)	–14.9 mL/minute
Statistical analysis indicated that telmisartan was not inferior to enalapril	
Secondary endpoints	
Effects of the two agents on any endpoint were not significantly different	

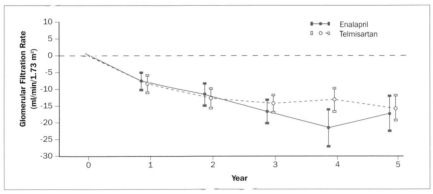

Figure 33. Changes from baseline in glomerular filtration rate. Reproduced with permission from the Massachusetts Medical Society.

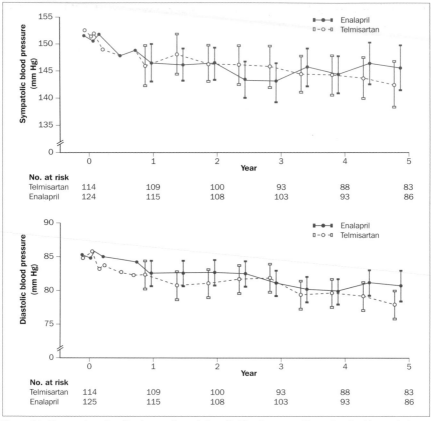

Figure 34. Changes from baseline in systolic and diastolic blood pressure. Reproduced with permission from the Massachusetts Medical Society.

Commentary

It is now well established that inhibitors of the renin–angiotensin system, which include ACE inhibitors and angiotensin-II receptor blockers, exert reno-protective effects in patients with diabetes and incipient or overt nephropathy. These two classes of agents block the renin–angiotensin system by different mechanisms.

This was the first long-term hard endpoint study to provide a comparison between these two approaches. When the protocol was written, enalapril was the gold standard ACE inhibitor and its comparator drug (telmisartan) was from a new class of agents, the angiotensin-II receptor blockers. The particular strength of this study was the 5-year follow-up period and the use of a hard endpoint measurement, ie, glomerular filtration rate – the gold standard measure of renal function.

The study demonstrated noninferiority of telmisartan versus enalapril in providing renal protection. Two extremely important findings from this study were:

- Renal function was almost completely stabilised beyond year 3 in both groups.

- There was extremely low overall mortality (5% in each group). Mortality was due to a cardiovascular event in only half of these patients.

The latter finding is particularly surprising, given that the expected mortality in this high-risk group (50% already had evidence of cardiovascular disease at enrolment into the study) was 35% at 5 years. This could be accounted for, in part, because of increased usage of drugs such as statins, aspirin and other antihypertensives, but also suggests a cardioprotective effect from inhibition of the renin–angiotensin system.

The study emphasises the importance of screening for and identifying nepropathy as early as possible in type 2 diabetes. This should be followed by aggressive intervention, which should include use of an inhibitor of the renin–angiotensin system.

Renoprotective effect of the angiotensin receptor antagonist irbesartan in patients with nephropathy due to type 2 diabetes

What does this trial tell us?

➤ Irbesartan is effective in protecting against the progress of nephropathy in type 2 diabetes

➤ This protection is independent of a reduction in blood pressure

Authors	Lewis EJ, Hunsicker LG, Clarke WR, et al, for the Collaborative Study Group
Reference	*N Engl J Med* 2001;345:851–60
Objective	To investigate whether the angiotensin-II receptor blocker irbesartan or the calcium-channel blocker amlodipine slows the progress of nephropathy in type 2 diabetes and whether any effect is independent of reduction in blood pressure
Methodology	Randomised controlled trial of irbesartan versus amlodipine or placebo
Drugs used	Irbesartan 300 mg/day, amlodipine 10 mg/day
Patients	1,715 hypertensive patients, aged 30–70 years, with nephropathy due to type 2 diabetes
Outcomes	The primary endpoint was a composite of doubling of baseline serum creatinine, development of end-stage renal disease or death from any cause. The secondary endpoint was a composite of cardiovascular outcomes
Analysis	Intention to treat
Follow-up	Mean 2.6 years

Results

Outcome	Adjusted relative risk	P value
Primary composite endpoint		
Irbesartan vs placebo	0.81	0.03
Amlodipine vs placebo	1.07	0.47
Irbesartan vs amlodipine	0.76	0.005
Doubling of serum creatinine		
Irbesartan vs placebo	0.71	0.009
Amlodipine vs placebo	1.15	0.24
Irbesartan vs amlodipine	0.61	<0.001
Cardiovascular composite		
Irbesartan vs placebo	0.91	0.40
Amlodipine vs placebo	0.88	0.27
Irbesartan vs amlodipine	1.03	0.78

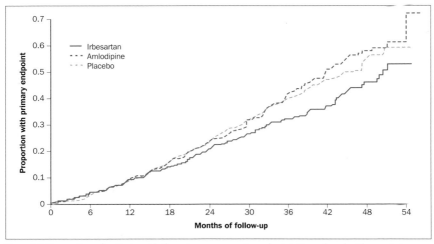

Figure 35. Proportion of patients with the primary composite endpoint. Reproduced with permission from the Massachusetts Medical Society.

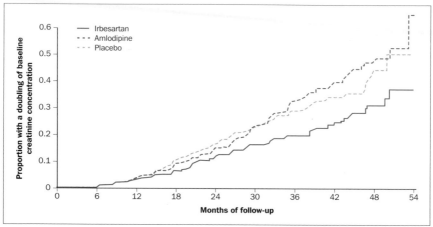

Figure 36. Proportion of patients with doubling of baseline serum creatinine concentration. Reproduced with permission from the Massachusetts Medical Society.

Commentary

This study was similar to the RENAAL trial described later (see p. 79). It used another angiotensin-II receptor blocker, irbesartan (RENAAL looked at losartan), in patients with type 2 diabetes and overt nephropathy. Again, the authors found evidence of renal protection with reduced progression of the disease process. However, there was no evidence for reversal of the disease process and no reduction in overall mortality or cardiovascular events.

It is clear from other studies that any renal involvement needs to be determined very early and treated aggressively, particularly with inhibitors of the renin–angiotensin system, including angiotensin-converting enzyme inhibitors or angiotensin-II receptor blockers.

The effect of irbesartan on the development of diabetic nephropathy in patients with type 2 diabetes

What does this trial tell us?

➤ The angiotensin-II receptor antagonist irbesartan is renoprotective in patients with type 2 diabetes and microalbuminuria

➤ This effect is independent of an irbesartan-induced reduction in blood pressure (BP)

Authors	Parving H-H, Lehnert H, Bröchner-Mortensen J, et al, for the Irbesartan in Patients with Type 2 Diabetes and Microalbuminuria Study Group
Reference	*N Engl J Med* 2001;345:870–8
Objective	To evaluate the renoprotective effect of irbesartan in hypertensive patients with type 2 diabetes and microalbuminuria
Methodology	Randomised controlled, double-blind study in 96 centres worldwide, comparing irbesartan with placebo
Drugs used	Irbesartan 150 mg/day or 300 mg/day
Patients	590 hypertensive patients with type 2 diabetes and persistent microalbuminuria
Outcomes	The primary endpoint was time to onset of diabetic nephropathy, defined by urinary albumin excretion rate. Secondary endpoints included HbA_{1c} and lowest arterial BP
Analysis	Intention to treat
Follow-up	2 years

Results

Endpoint	Placebo	Irbesartan 150 mg	Irbesartan 300 mg
Patients developing persistent albuminuria, n (%)	30 (14.9)	19 (9.7)	10 (5.2)
P value compared with placebo		0.08	<0.001
Average BP (mm Hg)	144/83	143/83*	141/83*
*For systolic BP between combined irbesartan groups compared with placebo: P=0.004			

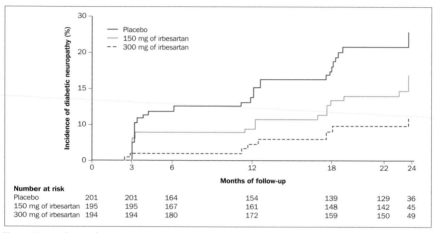

Figure 37. Incidence of progression to diabetic nephropathy. Difference between placebo group and irbesartan 300 mg group was significant by log-rank test (P<0.001). Reproduced with permission from the Massachusetts Medical Society.

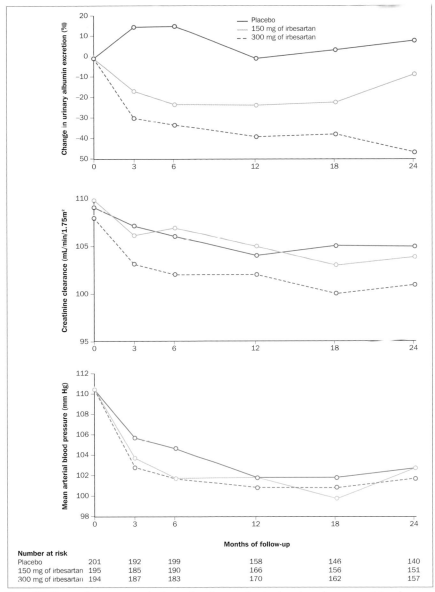

Figure 38. Geometric mean rates of urinary albumin excretion (**top**), estimated mean creatinine clearance (**middle**) and trough mean arterial blood pressure (**bottom**). Average urinary albumin excretion rate was significantly reduced in both irbesartan groups (*P*<0.001). Blood pressure was significantly reduced in the irbesartan 300 mg group compared with placebo (*P*=0.005). Reproduced with permission from the Massachusetts Medical Society.

Commentary

Diabetic nephropathy is the single most common reason for renal failure and the leading cause for dialysis in many countries, including western Europe and the US. The finding of microalbuminuria, an albumin excretion rate above the normal range but below the level of standard stick test detection, is predictive of both later development of overt proteinuria/diabetic nephropathy and increased cardiovascular risk.

In this study, patients with microalbuminuria (incipient nephropathy), hypertension and type 2 diabetes were randomised to receive the angiotensin-II receptor blocker irbesartan or placebo. This was not a hypertension trial and attempts were made to achieve similar BP control in both arms of the study by use of other antihypertensives. In the 2-year follow-up, there was evidence for significant protection – ie, reduced progression from incipient to overt nephropathy with the angiotensin-II receptor blocker compared with placebo. There also appeared to be a profound dose relationship: irbesartan 300 mg/day was superior to 150 mg/day in slowing such progression.

This study emphasises the importance of early screening for diabetic renal disease and very active intervention (see also the BENEDICT study, p. 64). This should always include an inhibitor of the renin–angiotensin system.

Effects of losartan on renal and cardiovascular outcomes in patients with type 2 diabetes and nephropathy

What does this trial tell us?

➤ Losartan confers significant renal benefits in patients with type 2 diabetes and nephropathy

➤ The treatment is generally well tolerated

Authors	Brenner BM, Cooper ME, de Zeeuw D, et al, for the Reduction of Endpoints in NIDDM with the Angiotensin-II Antagonist Losartan (RENAAL) Study Investigators
Reference	*N Engl J Med* 2001;345:861–9
Objective	To assess the effects of the angiotensin-II receptor antagonist losartan in patients with type 2 diabetes and nephropathy
Methodology	Randomised, double-blind study comparing losartan with placebo, both in addition to conventional antihypertensive treatment
Drugs used	Losartan 50–100 mg/day and conventional antihypertensive treatment (calcium-channel blockers, diuretics, alpha-blockers, beta-blockers, centrally acting agents); doses depended on trough blood pressure
Patients	1,513 patients, aged 31–70 years, with type 2 diabetes and nephropathy, diagnosed on the basis of urinary albumin and serum creatinine levels
Outcomes	The primary endpoint was a composite of doubled baseline serum creatinine, end-stage renal disease and death. Secondary endpoints included a composite of morbidity and mortality from cardiovascular causes
Analysis	Intention to treat
Follow-up	Mean 3.4 years

Results

Incidence of the primary composite renal endpoint and its components				
Endpoint	Losartan group, n (%)	Placebo group, n (%)	P value	Risk reduction, %
Primary composite	327 (43.5)	359 (47.1)	0.02	16
Doubled serum creatinine	162 (21.6)	198 (26.0)	0.006	25
End-stage renal disease	147 (19.6)	194 (25.5)	0.002	28
Death	158 (21.0)	155 (20.3)	0.88	-2
End-stage renal disease or death	255 (34.0)	300 (39.4)	0.01	20

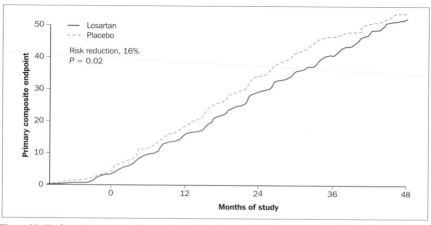

Figure 39. Kaplan–Meier curves of percentages of patients with the primary composite endpoint. Reproduced with permission from the Massachusetts Medical Society.

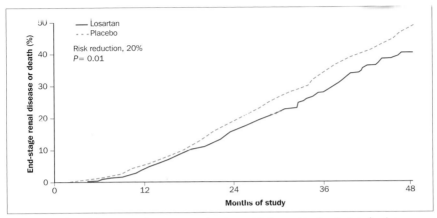

Figure 40. Kaplan–Meier curves of percentages of patients with the combined endpoint of end-stage renal disease or death. Reproduced with permission from the Massachusetts Medical Society.

Commentary

Diabetes is now the single most common reason for the development of chronic renal failure and need for dialysis in many countries in the world, including western Europe and the US. Many studies have looked at preventing or slowing the progression of kidney disease in diabetic patients. In this study, the effect of the angiotensin-II receptor antagonist losartan was examined in patients with type 2 diabetes and overt nephropathy. Evidence of renal protection was found, with reduced progression of the primary endpoint.

Although there was evidence of renal benefit, there was no evidence for reversal of the disease process and no reduction in overall mortality or cardiovascular events. It is clear from other studies that any renal involvement needs to be determined very early and treated aggressively, particularly with inhibitors of the renin–angiotensin system, including angiotensin-converting enzyme inhibitors and angiotensin-II receptor blockers.

Randomised controlled trial of dual blockade of renin–angiotensin system in patients with hypertension, microalbuminuria and non-insulin dependent diabetes: the candesartan and lisinopril microalbuminuria (CALM) study

What does this trial tell us?

➤ Candesartan 16 mg/day is as effective as lisinopril 20 mg/day in reducing blood pressure (BP) and microalbuminuria in hypertensive patients with type 2 diabetes

➤ Combination treatment is more effective than monotherapy in reducing BP, and is well tolerated

Authors	Mogensen CE, Neldam S, Tikkanen I, et al, for the CALM Study Group
Reference	*BMJ* 2000;321:1440–4
Objective	To assess and compare the effects of the angiotensin-II type 1 (AT1) receptor blocker candesartan or the angiotensin-converting enzyme (ACE) inhibitor lisinopril, or both, in patients with microalbuminuria, hypertension and type 2 diabetes
Methodology	Prospective, randomised, parallel-group, double-blind study, with 4-week placebo run-in and 12 weeks of monotherapy with candesartan or lisinopril followed by 12 weeks of monotherapy or combination treatment
Drugs used	Candesartan 16 mg/day, lisinopril 20 mg/day
Patients	199 patients, aged 30–75 years, with type 2 diabetes, microalbuminuria assessed by urinary albumin:creatinine ratio and diastolic BP ≥90–100 mm Hg
Outcomes	Primary endpoints were urinary albumin:creatinine ratio and BP. Secondary endpoints included HbA_{1c} and serum creatinine levels
Analysis	Intention to treat, last value carried forward
Follow-up	24 weeks

Results

Adjusted mean reductions in BP and urinary albumin:creatinine ratio from baseline to 24 weeks					
Endpoint	Candesartan	Lisinopril	Combination	Adjusted mean difference	
				Combination vs candesartan	Combination vs lisinopril
Sitting diastolic BP (mm Hg)	10.4 (P<0.001)	10.7 (P<0.001)	16.3 (P<0.001)	5.9 (P=0.003)	5.6 (P=0.005)
Sitting systolic BP (mm Hg)	14.1 (P<0.001)	16.7 (P<0.001)	25.3 (P<0.001)	11.2 (P=0.002)	8.6 (P=0.02)
Urinary albumin: creatinine ratio (%)	24 (P=0.05)	39 (P<0.001)	50 (P<0.001)	34 (P=0.004)	18 (P>0.20)

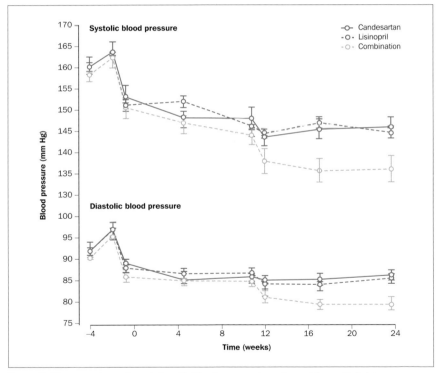

Figure 41. Mean seated systolic and diastolic blood pressures in patients with type 2 diabetes, hypertension and microalbuminuria before and during treatment with candesartan, lisinopril or combination therapy. Reproduced with permission from BMJ Publishing.

Commentary

Although it has been well reported that both ACE inhibitors and AT1 receptor blockers are associated with renal protection in type 2 diabetes, a combination of these agents might have even more profound benefits – they inhibit the renin–angiotensin system via different mechanisms, and might therefore have additive effects.

This short-term study compared the effects of an ACE inhibitor versus an AT1 receptor blocker versus a combination of the two in patients with microalbuminuria, hypertension and type 2 diabetes. The authors found the AT1 receptor blocker to be as effective as the ACE inhibitor in reducing BP and microalbuminuria in this cohort – importantly, the combination treatment was more effective than monotherapy in reducing BP and probably proteinuria than each agent alone.

This was only a short-term study, and further work needs to be done in this area. In the meantime, given the additive effect on BP, it would seem reasonable to allow both of these classes of agents to be used together in the management of raised BP. Such a combination should normally be tried if there is an insufficient response to traditional combinations, which would normally include an inhibitor of the renin–angiotensin system with a diuretic and calcium-channel blocker.

Development and progression of nephropathy in type 2 diabetes: the United Kingdom Prospective Diabetes Study (UKPDS 64)

What does this trial tell us?

➤ The proportion of patients with type 2 diabetes who develop microalbuminuria is substantial, with one-quarter affected by 10 years from diagnosis

➤ Relatively fewer patients develop macroalbuminuria, but in those who do, the death rate exceeds the rate of progression to worse nephropathy

Authors	Adler, AI, Stevens, RJ, Manley, SE, et al, for the UKPDS Group
Reference	*Kidney Int* 2003;63:225–32
Objective	To investigate the development and progression of micro- to macroalbuminuria in patients with type 2 diabetes
Methodology	Analysis of observed and modelled data from UKPDS, measuring the annual probability of transition of micro- and macroalbuminuria from stage to stage and risk of death from all-cause or cardiovascular causes
Patients	5,097 patients, aged 25–65 years, with newly diagnosed type 2 diabetes
Outcomes	Nephropathy progression, elevated plasma creatinine, renal replacement therapy and death
Analysis	Calculation of annual transition probabilities; use of Mantel–Haenszel test to investigate the hypothesis that risk of cardiovascular death increases with worsening nephropathy; use of Markov model to estimate the prevalence beyond years of observation
Follow-up	15 years

Results

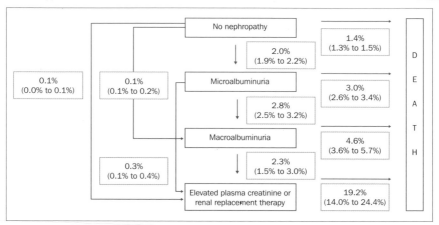

Figure 42. Annual transition rates through the stages of nephropathy and to death from any cause. Reproduced with permission from the International Society of Nephrology.

Commentary

This study from the UKPDS Group was an analysis of observed and model data that measured the annual probability of transition of micro- and microalbuminuria from stage to stage, and then related this to risk of death from all causes or cardiovascular causes. The findings support other studies that have demonstrated increased mortality (particularly from cardiovascular disease) in association with increased urinary albumin excretion. Microalbuminuria was found to be associated with a reduced likelihood of survival at 10 years, with even worse survival rates once macroalbuminuria is present.

The authors found the prevalence of microalbuminuria to be substantial, although the transition rate to macroalbuminuria was relatively low. For those who developed macroalbuminuria, death ensued in the majority before the development of overt chronic renal failure.

Retinopathy

Microaneurysms in the development of diabetic retinopathy (UKPDS 42)

What does this trial tell us?

➤ Microaneurysms (MAs) are a significant diabetic symptom, with a high risk of progression to severe retinopathy

➤ Even one or two MAs in an eye should not be disregarded

➤ Patients with four or more MAs are at risk of developing sight-threatening retinopathy

Authors	Kohner EM, Stratton IM, Aldington SJ, et al, for the UK Prospective Diabetes Study (UKPDS) Group
Reference	*Diabetologia* 1999;42:1107–12
Objective	To determine whether MAs, in the absence of other lesions, have a predictive role in the progression of diabetic retinopathy in type 2 diabetes
Methodology	Hyperglycaemic but otherwise symptom-free patients were randomly allocated to diet alone or treatment with hypoglycaemic medication
Drugs used	Insulin, oral hypoglycaemics; dose as clinically indicated
Patients	5,102 patients with type 2 diabetes; 3,569 had retinal photographs taken at entry
Outcomes	Progression of retinopathy, as assessed by ophthalmoscopy and retinal photographs; visual acuity
Analysis	Chi-squared statistics to determine trend in retinopathy severity relative to numbers of MAs
Follow-up	Up to 12 years (414 patients)

Results

Retinopathy level at 6 years in those without MAs at 3 years			
No. of MAs at entry	No. retinopathy, n (%)	MAs only, n (%)	More severe retinopathy, n (%)
0	600 (67.0)	196 (21.9)	100 (11.1)
1	69 (56.1)	38 (30.9)	16 (13.0)
2	24 (55.8)	11 (25.6)	8 (18.6)
3	11 (64.7)	5 (29.4)	1 (5.9)
4	5 (55.5)	3 (33.3)	1 (11.1)
≥5	5 (62.5)	1 (12.5)	2 (25.0)
Mantel–Haenszel chi-squared for trend 0.936, P=0.333			

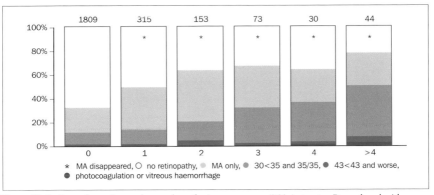

Figure 43. Retinopathy at 3 years by number of microaneurysms (MAs) at entry. Reproduced with permission from Springer-Verlag.

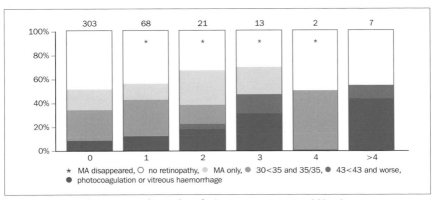

Figure 44. Retinopathy at 12 years by number of microaneurysms at entry. MA: microaneurysm. Reproduced with permission from Springer-Verlag.

Commentary

Traditional teaching on the prognosis of diabetic retinopathy suggested that just a few MAs are of little clinical significance. This UKPDS paper suggested otherwise, and has led to changes in clinical practice. The authors had retinal photography from around three quarters of the original UKPDS cohort, and used this data to look at the progress of retinopathy over time. The principal finding was that MAs are associated with a higher risk of progression to severe retinopathy, even when allowing for other retinal lesions. In particular, patients with four or more MAs are at risk of developing sight-threatening retinopathy.

This paper emphasises the importance of regular retinal screening using accredited methods (today, by digital retinal photography) and the realisation of the importance of various retinal lesions, including MAs, as a predictor of risk for progression to sight-threatening retinopathy.

Risks of progression of retinopathy and vision loss related to tight blood pressure control in type 2 diabetes mellitus (UKPDS 69)

What does this trial tell us?

➤ High blood pressure (BP) is detrimental to each aspect of diabetic retinopathy

➤ A tight BP control policy reduces the risk of clinical complications from eye disease

Authors	Matthews DR, Stratton IM, Aldington SJ, et al, for the UK Prospective Diabetes Study (UKPDS) Group
Reference	*Arch Ophthalmol* 2004;122:1631–40
Objective	To determine the relationship between BP control and diabetic retinopathy in patients with type 2 diabetes
Methodology	Randomised controlled trial comparing tight BP control (angiotensin-converting enzyme inhibitor or beta-blockers, aiming for <150/85 mm Hg) with less tight control (aiming for <180/105 mm Hg)
Drugs used	Captopril 25–50 mg twice daily, atenolol 50–100 mg twice daily
Patients	1,148 hypertensive patients with type 2 diabetes (mean BP 160/94 mm Hg): 758 allocated to tight BP control and 390 to less tight control
Outcomes	Deterioration of retinopathy as assessed by a modified Early Treatment Diabetic Retinopathy (ETDRS) final scale, photocoagulation, vitreous haemorrhage, cataract extraction, specific lesions such as hard exudates, visual acuity
Analysis	Intention to treat
Follow-up	7.5 years

Results

Relative risk of 2-step or worse retinal deterioration in patients randomised to the tight (TBP) and less tight (LTBP) control groups				
Time after randomisation (years)	No. (%) of patients with ≥ 2-step deterioration		Relative risk for intensive policy	P value
	TBP group	LTBP group		
1.5	93 (20.2)	56 (23.1)	0.88	0.38
4.5	113 (27.5)	76 (36.7)	0.75	0.019
7.5	102 (34.0)	78 (51.3)	0.66	0.001
Prevalence of blindness from all causes in the TBP and LTBP control groups				
Time after randomisation (years)	No. of events (eg, cataract, diabetic maculopathy)		Relative risk for intensive policy	P value
	TBP group	LTBP group		
7.5	758	390	0.76	0.46

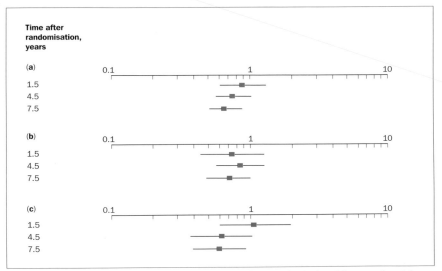

Figure 45. Relative risk of 2-step or worse deterioration in those randomised to tight versus less tight blood pressure control. (a) Overall randomisation. (b) No retinopathy at randomisation. (c) Any retinopathy at randomisation. Reproduced with permission from the American Medical Association.

Commentary

Although it is now well established that poor glycaemic control is a major risk factor for the development or progression of diabetic microvascular disease, including retinopathy, it is only in more recent years that the importance of BP has been recognised. It is perhaps surprising that although hypertension has been a recognised risk factor for cardiovascular disease for many years, the possibility that it might also impact on retinopathy is a much newer concept.

This study from the UKPDS Group clearly showed that raised BP has a detrimental effect on each aspect of diabetic retinopathy, and that tightening BP control reduces the risk of progression of retinopathy. This study supports a whole range of other studies, all of which point to hypertension as a significant risk factor in the development and progression of retinopathy. It emphasises the importance of tight BP control, not only to reduce the risk of cardiovascular disease, but also to reduce the risk of microvascular disease.

Erectile Dysfunction

Sildenafil citrate for the treatment of erectile dysfunction in men with type II diabetes mellitus

What does this trial tell us?

➤ Sildenafil is effective in improving erectile dysfunction in men with type 2 diabetes, even in those with poor glycaemic control and complications

➤ Sildenafil is well tolerated in this patient group

Authors	Boulton AJM, Selam J-L, Sweeney M, Ziegler D
Reference	*Diabetologia* 2001;44:1296–301
Objective	To evaluate the effects of sildenafil in men with type 2 diabetes and erectile dysfunction
Methodology	Double-blind, placebo-controlled, 12-week trial of sildenafil versus placebo
Drugs used	Sildenafil citrate 50 mg/day initially, adjusted to 25 mg or 100 mg depending on efficacy and tolerability
Patients	219 male patients, mean age 59 years, with type 2 diabetes and erectile dysfunction as assessed by the International Index of Erectile Function (IIEF, score range 0–5)
Outcomes	Primary endpoints were achieving and maintaining an erection as assessed by the IIEF. Secondary endpoints included life satisfaction and global efficacy
Analysis	Intention to treat; efficacy variables analysed by ANCOVA
Follow-up	12 weeks

Results

Outcome	Baseline	Placebo	Sildenafil
IIEF Q3 (achieving erection), mean score	1.77	1.86	3.42 (P<0.0001 vs placebo)
IIEF Q4 (maintaining erection), mean score	1.49	1.84	3.35 (P<0.0001 vs placebo)
IIEF Qs1–5,15 (erectile function domain), mean score	10.4	11.5	20.4 (P<0.0001 vs placebo)
Successful attempts, estimated %	13.8	14.4	58.8 (P<0.0001 vs placebo)
Sexual life satisfaction, Life Satisfaction Checklist	–	2.55	3.79 (P<0.0001 vs placebo)

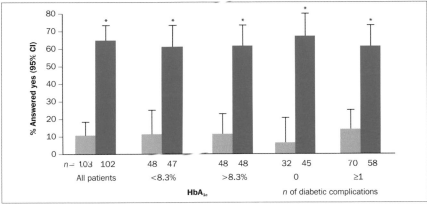

Figure 46. After 12 weeks of treatment, percentage of patients answering "yes" to the question: "Did treatment improve your erections?" (Sildenafil compared with placebo: $P<0.0001$). Reproduced with permission from Springer-Verlag.

Commentary

Around 50% of diabetic men complain of erectile dysfunction. Prior to the first decade of the new millennium, the mainstay of treatment was either local injection of appropriate agents, vacuum pump devices or implantable devices. The advent of sildenafil heralded a revolution in the management of erectile dysfunction. Since then, several similar agents have also come onto the market.

In this study, the authors evaluated the effects of sildenafil in men with type 2 diabetes and erectile dysfunction. Sildenafil was found to be effective in improving such dysfunction in men with type 2 diabetes, even if there was poor glycaemic control and/or complications, and was generally well tolerated. This agent can be prescribed in primary care and is now widely available and used.

97

Prevention
of Diabetes

Reduction in the incidence of type 2 diabetes with lifestyle intervention or metformin

What does this trial tell us?

➤ Lifestyle changes and metformin both reduce the incidence of diabetes in subjects at high risk

➤ Lifestyle intervention is significantly more effective than metformin

Authors	Diabetes Prevention Program Research Group
Reference	*N Engl J Med* 2002;346:393–403
Objective	To investigate whether modification of lifestyle risk factors or administration of metformin would prevent or delay development of diabetes in subjects at high risk
Methodology	Randomised controlled trial comparing standard lifestyle recommendations plus metformin, standard lifestyle recommendations plus placebo and an intensive lifestyle-modification programme (goals of 7% weight loss and ≥150 minutes physical activity/week)
Drugs used	Metformin 850 mg twice daily
Patients	3,234 non-diabetic patients, mean age 51 years, with elevated fasting and post-load plasma glucose concentrations
Outcomes	The primary outcome was diabetes, diagnosed by American Diabetic Association criteria. Secondary outcomes included leisure physical activity, body weight and daily caloric intake
Analysis	Intention to treat
Follow-up	Average 2.8 years

Results

Incidence of diabetes			
Group	Placebo	Metformin	Lifestyle
Incidence (cases per 100 person-years)	11.0	7.8	4.8
	Lifestyle vs placebo	Metformin vs placebo	Lifestyle vs metformin
Risk reduction	58%*	31%*	39%*
*Statistically significant according to group-sequential log-rank test			

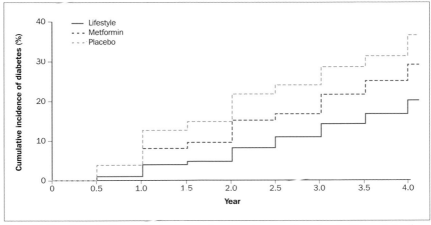

Figure 47. Cumulative incidence of diabetes according to study group. Reproduced with permission from the Massachusetts Medical Society.

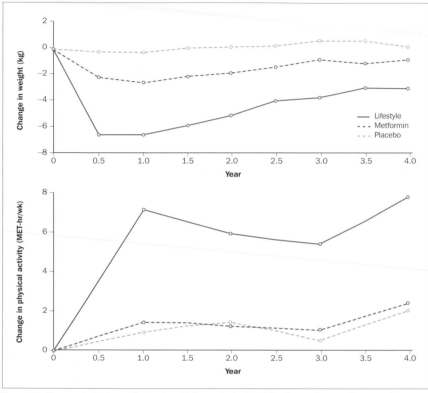

Figure 48. Changes in body weight (**top**) and leisure physical activity (**bottom**) according to study group. Reproduced with permission from the Massachusetts Medical Society.

Commentary

This major study investigated whether modification of lifestyle risk factors (diet and exercise) or administration of metformin would prevent or delay the development of diabetes in high-risk individuals (ie, those with impaired glucose tolerance). Compared with placebo over an almost 3-year mean period of follow-up, there was a 58% risk reduction in conversion to type 2 diabetes in the lifestyle group and a 31% risk reduction in the metformin group.

This trial emphasises the value of lifestyle interventions in the prevention or slowing of progression of type 2 diabetes in high-risk individuals. Interestingly, lifestyle was more effective than metformin treatment, indicating that lifestyle intervention should be the primary approach to prevention of type 2 diabetes. One might add that where lifestyle advice will not or cannot be followed, metformin offers a pharmacotherapeutic option, which might exert its beneficial effects through improved insulin sensitivity. This remains a controversial area and needs further study.

Prevention of type 2 diabetes mellitus by changes in lifestyle among subjects with impaired glucose tolerance

What does this trial tell us?

➤ The onset of type 2 diabetes can be prevented by changes in the lifestyle of high-risk subjects

➤ Lifestyle changes may reduce the risk of type 2 diabetes in this group of patients by 58% or more

Authors	Tuomilehto J, Lindström J, Eriksson JG, et al, for the Finnish Diabetes Prevention Study Group
Reference	*N Engl J Med* 2001;344:1343–50
Objective	To investigate whether type 2 diabetes can be prevented by interventions that affect the lifestyles of subjects at high risk for the disorder
Methodology	Randomised controlled study of individualised intervention (counselling aimed at reducing weight, total intake of fat and intake of saturated fat, and increasing intake of fibre and physical activity) versus general diet and exercise advice
Patients	522 middle-aged, overweight subjects with impaired glucose tolerance
Outcomes	Diabetes as defined by World Health Organization criteria (fasting plasma glucose ≤140 mg/dL, or plasma glucose ≤200 mg/dL at 2 hours after oral glucose challenge)
Analysis	Intention to treat. Difference between groups in incidence of diabetes tested by means of two-sided log-rank test
Follow-up	Mean 3.2 years

Results

Success in achieving intervention goals by 1 year, according to treatment group			
Goal	Intervention group, %	Control group, %	P value
Weight reduction >5%	43	13	0.001
Fat intake <30% of energy intake	47	26	0.001
Saturated fat intake <10% of energy intake	26	11	0.001
Fibre intake ≥ 15 g/1,000 kcal	25	12	0.001
Exercise >4 hours/week	86	71	0.001

Risk of diabetes			
Intervention group, % cumulative incidence after 4 years	Control group, % cumulative incidence after 4 years	% Risk reduction during trial	P value for risk reduction during trial
11	23	58	<0.001

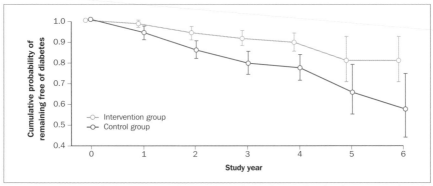

Figure 49. Proportion of subjects without diabetes during the trial. Reproduced with permission from the Massachusetts Medical Society.

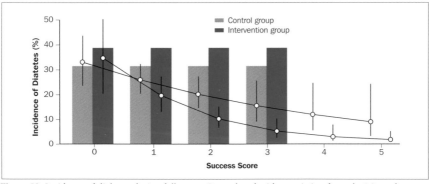

Figure 50. Incidence of diabetes during follow-up. Reproduced with permission from the Massachusetts Medical Society.

Commentary

Type 2 diabetes has reached epidemic proportions in many parts of the world. This epidemic is driven by obesity, which is now a major public health problem in both the developed and developing worlds.

In this important study, the investigators aimed to determine whether type 2 diabetes could be prevented or progression slowed by lifestyle measures, including diet and exercise advice. Over a mean 3.2 years of follow-up, there was significantly greater weight reduction in the intervention group, and more exercise was taken. After 4 years, the cumulative incidence of type 2 diabetes demonstrated a 58% risk reduction in the active treatment group. This study emphasises the important point that lifestyle measures can help slow progression to type 2 diabetes in high-risk individuals. What the trial could not tell us was whether this was *slowing of progression* or *absolute prevention* of the disease.

Ramipril and the development of diabetes

What does this trial tell us?

➤ Ramipril reduces the risk of new diagnoses of diabetes in high-risk individuals

➤ As these results have major clinical and public health implications, they require prospective confirmation

Authors	Yusuf S, Gerstein H, Hoogwerf B, et al, for the Heart Outcomes Prevention Evaluation (HOPE) Study Investigators
Reference	*JAMA* 2001;286:1882–5
Objective	To investigate the effectiveness of the angiotensin-converting enzyme (ACE) inhibitor ramipril in preventing diabetes in high-risk patients
Methodology	Follow-up of the randomised, controlled, HOPE trial, comparing ramipril with placebo (*Lancet* 2000;255:253–9)
Drugs used	Ramipril up to 10 mg/day
Patients	5,720 patients, aged >55 years, without known diabetes but with vascular disease (eg, coronary heart disease, hypertension)
Outcomes	The primary endpoint was diagnosis of diabetes, assessed every 6 months. Secondary endpoints included HbA_{1c} level and death from any cause
Analysis	Intention to treat
Follow-up	Mean 4.5 years

Results

Effect of ramipril on the development of new diabetes stratified by the occurrence of specific events (eg, cardiovascular events)				
Variables	Ramipril, n (%)	Placebo, n (%)	Relative risk	P value
With primary event	9 (2.4)	26 (5.5)	0.46	0.04
No primary event	93 (3.8)	129 (5.4)	0.69	0.007
With new microalbuminuria or overt nephropathy	20 (5.6)	36 (8.4)	0.65	0.12
No new microalbuminuria or overt nephropathy	82 (3.3)	119 (4.9)	0.67	0.005

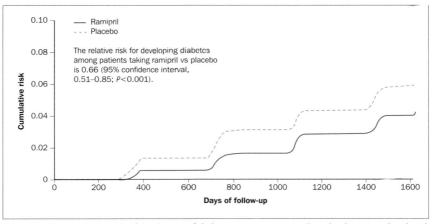

Figure 51. The cumulative risk of developing of diabetes over time: ramipril vs placebo. Reproduced with permission from the American Medical Association.

	Ramipril		Placebo		Interaction
	Patients	No. (%) with diabetes	Patients	No. (%) with diabetes	P value
Waist–hip ratio >0.93	1445	63 (4.4)	1508	104 (6.9)	
Waist–hip ratio ≤ 0.93	1392	39 (2.8)	1375	51 (3.7)	0.46
Body mass index >27.7 kg/m²	1095	63 (5.8)	1146	94 (8.2)	
Body mass index ≤ 27.7 kg/m²	1742	39 (2.2)	1737	61 (3.5)	0.79
With hypertension	1167	49 (4.2)	1192	76 (6.4)	
Without hypertension	1670	53 (3.2)	1691	79 (4.7)	0.86
With microalbuminuria	402	17 (4.2)	421	35 (8.3)	
Without microalbuminuria	2435	85 (3.5)	2462	120 (4.9)	0.26
Taking beta-blocker	1310	52 (4.0)	1348	66 (4.9)	
Not taking beta-blocker	1527	50 (3.3)	1535	89 (5.8)	0.15
Taking diuretics	363	18 (5.0)	356	28 (7.9)	
Not taking diuretics	2474	84 (3.4)	2527	127 (5.0)	0.86

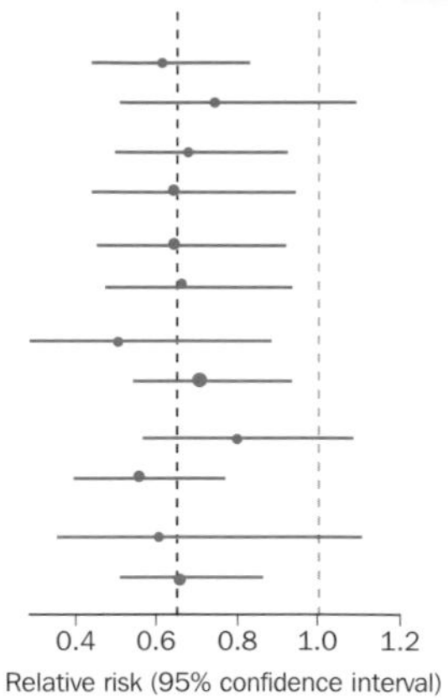

0.4   0.6   0.8   1.0   1.2
Relative risk (95% confidence interval)

Waist–hip ratio and body mass index are subdivided above and below the median. The size of the boxes are proportionate to the number of patients. Dashed line indicates the average treatment effect; dotted line, relative risk equal to 1.

Figure 52. Effect of ramipril in preventing diabetes in subgroups defined at randomisation. Reproduced with permission from the American Medical Association.

Commentary

This study arose from the HOPE trial, which compared ramipril with placebo in individuals with high cardiovascular risk, including diabetic patients. Of almost 6,000 patients without known diabetes and with established vascular disease, the use of ramipril was associated with approximately 33% reduced risk of progression to type 2 diabetes. This study has since been supported by other trials of inhibitors of the renin–angiotensin system, which have shown similar benefits in reducing the risk of development of type 2 diabetes.

The mechanism of this effect, and indeed whether it is a true effect, is still undetermined, although there is some evidence that these agents improve insulin resistance. Further work is ongoing in this area.

Multifactorial Interventions

Multifactorial intervention and cardiovascular disease in patients with type 2 diabetes

What does this trial tell us?

➤ Intensive intervention aimed at multiple risk factors in type 2 diabetes with microalbuminuria reduces the risk of cardiovascular and microvascular events by about 50%

Authors	Gæde P, Vedel P, Larsen N, et al
Reference	N Engl J Med 2003;348:383–93
Objective	To compare the effect of a targeted, intensified, multifactorial intervention with that of conventional treatment on modifiable risk factors for cardiovascular disease in patients with type 2 diabetes and microalbuminuria
Methodology	Open, parallel trial with patients randomised to intensive treatment (behaviour modification and pharmacological therapy that targeted hyperglycaemia, hypertension, dyslipidaemia and microalbuminuria) or conventional treatment
Drugs used	Targeted medications (eg, insulin, antihypertensives) as clinically required, together with aspirin 150 mg/day for secondary prevention of cardiovascular disease in both groups. All patients were also given vitamin supplements
Patients	160 patients, mean age 55.1 years, with type 2 diabetes and persistent microalbuminuria
Outcomes	The primary endpoint was a composite of death from cardiovascular causes, non-fatal myocardial infarction, non-fatal stroke, revascularisation and amputation. Secondary endpoints included incidence of diabetic nephropathy and development or progression of diabetic nephropathy or neuropathy
Analysis	Intention to treat
Follow-up	Mean 7.8 years

Results

Main changes in clinical, behavioural and biochemical variables at end of study (means)			
Variable	Conventional therapy	Intensive therapy	P value
Systolic blood pressure (mm Hg)	−3	−14	<0.001
Diastolic blood pressure (mm Hg)	−8	−12	0.006
Fat (% of energy intake)	−6.8	−10.4	<0.001
Saturated fatty acids (% of energy intake)	−4.4	−6.9	<0.001
Fasting plasma glucose (mg/dL)	−18	−52	<0.001
HbA$_{1c}$ (%)	0.2	−0.5	<0.001
Fasting serum triglycerides (mg/dL)	9	−41	0.015
Fasting serum total cholesterol (mg/dL)	−3	−50	<0.001
Fasting serum low-density lipoprotein cholesterol (mg/dL)	−13	−47	<0.001
Urinary albumin excretion (mmol/24 hours)	30	−20	0.007

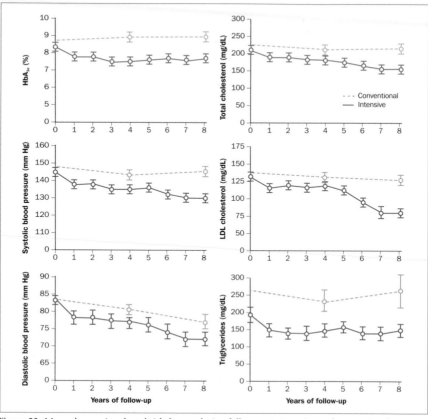

Figure 53. Mean changes in selected risk factors during follow-up in intensive and conventional therapy groups. LDL: low-density lipoprotein. Reproduced with permission from the Massachusetts Medical Society.

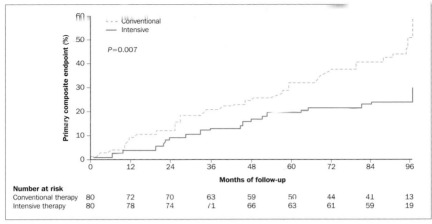

Number at risk

Conventional therapy	80	72	70	63	59	50	44	41	13
Intensive therapy	80	78	74	71	66	63	61	59	19

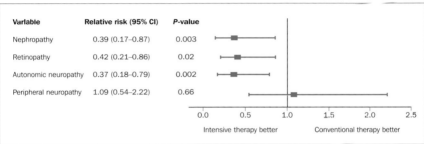

Figure 54. Kaplan–Meier estimates of the composite cardiovascular endpoint (**top**) and relative risks of the secondary endpoints at a mean of 7.8 years (**bottom**). CI: confidence interval. Reproduced with permission from the Massachusetts Medical Society.

Commentary

This was the first study to attempt to comprehensively investigate the outcomes from multiple cardiovascular risk factor interventions in higher-risk type 2 diabetic patients with persistent microalbuminuria. The study has gained an extremely high profile, although study numbers (160 patients) were relatively low. The authors compared the effect of a targeted, intensified, multifactorial intervention with that of conventional treatment on modifiable risk factors for cardiovascular disease.

This study demonstrated clear benefits of intensive intervention, reducing the risk of cardiovascular and microvascular events by around 50%. The trial demonstrated profound improvements in both systolic and diastolic blood pressure, and in lipid profile, in the intensive group compared with the conventional therapy group. This was associated with a highly significant reduction in both the primary and secondary endpoints.

113

Although greater reductions in HbA_{1c} were demonstrated in the intensively treated group, the authors found it extremely difficult to reach the HbA_{1c} target, testifying to the difficulty in achieving good glycaemic control. Benefits on blood pressure reduction and improvement in the lipid profile were considerably more profound.

Another finding was the lack of difference between the two groups in development of peripheral neuropathy (but, interestingly, not autonomic neuropathy, where the risk was significantly reduced by intensive treatment).

Management

Rosiglitazone short-term monotherapy lowers fasting and post-prandial glucose in patients with type II diabetes

What does this trial tell us?

➤ In patients with type 2 diabetes, rosiglitazone (RSG) twice daily significantly reduces fasting and postprandial glucose concentrations, C peptide, insulin and non-esterified fatty acids

➤ RSG is safe and well-tolerated

➤ The data suggest that 4 mg twice daily should be the maximum clinical dose

Authors	Raskin P, Rappaport EB, Cole ST, et al
Reference	*Diabetologia* 2000;43:278–84
Objective	To compare the short-term efficacy, safety and tolerability of RSG and placebo in type 2 diabetes
Methodology	Multicentre, randomised, double-blind, placebo-controlled 8-week trial
Drugs used	RSG (a thiazolidinedione, a group of drugs that reduce insulin resistance) 2, 4 or 6 mg twice daily
Patients	303 patients, aged 40–80 years, with type 2 diabetes who did not require insulin therapy
Outcomes	Glycaemic control (fasting plasma glucose), HbA_{1c}, insulin, C-peptide, fasting blood lipids
Analysis	Intention to treat, last observation carried forward
Follow-up	8 weeks

Results

Outcome	Placebo	RSG 2 mg bd	RSG 4 mg bd
Fasting plasma glucose			
Baseline	12.7	12.7	12.8
Week 4	13.7	11.4	10.9
Week 8	13.8	10.7	10.4
Significance of change from baseline to week 8	$P=0.0004$	$P<0.0001$	$P<0.0001$
HDL cholesterol (mmol/L)			
Baseline	1.19	1.13	1.17
Week 8	1.24	1.20	1.25
LDL cholesterol (mmol/L)			
Baseline	3.4	3.2	3.3
Week 8	3.4	3.7*	3.7*
Non-esterified fatty acids (mmol/L)			
Baseline	0.63	0.59	0.62
Week 8	0.70	0.49*	0.45*

HDL: high-density lipoprotein; LDL: low-density lipoprotein. *Significant difference from placebo

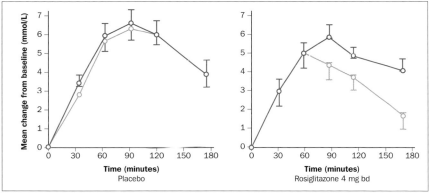

Figure 55. Reduction by rosiglitazone of fasting plasma glucose concentrations after 8 weeks of treatment. All values from the rosiglitazone-treated group were significantly different from placebo ($P<0.0001$). Error bars are standard deviations. Reproduced with permission from Springer-Verlag.

117

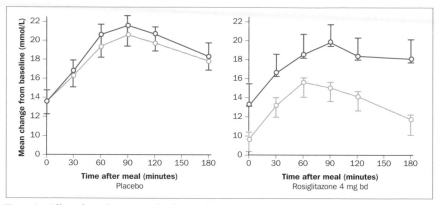

Figure 56. Effect of rosiglitazone or placebo on plasma glucose concentrations after a standard meal. Error bars represent standard errors. Reproduced with permission from Springer-Verlag.

Commentary

This early study of the use of a glitazone, RSG, in patients with type 2 diabetes showed that, when used as a monotherapy, this agent lowers fasting and postprandial glucose in patients with type 2 diabetes. This was associated with reductions in C-peptide and insulin (suggesting increased insulin sensitivity) and non-esterified fatty acids. The authors found RSG to be safe and well tolerated. Glitazones have since come into common usage, both as a monotherapy and as combination therapy in the management of type 2 diabetes.

Less hypoglycemia with insulin glargine in intensive insulin therapy for type 1 diabetes

What does this trial tell us?

➤ In intensive therapy for type 1 diabetes, lower fasting blood glucose levels (FGB) with fewer episodes of hypoglycaemia can be achieved with insulin glargine compared with human NPH insulin

➤ Insulin glargine has a good safety profile and is well tolerated

Authors	Ratner RE, Hirsch IB, Neifing JL, et al, for the US Study Group of Insulin Glargine in Type 1 Diabetes
Reference	*Diabetes Care* 2000;23:639–43
Objective	To compare the biosynthetic analogue insulin glargine with NPH human insulin in patients with type 1 diabetes who had been previously treated with multiple daily injections of NPH insulin and regular insulin
Methodology	Multicentre, randomised, parallel-group study in which patients received regular insulin plus either insulin glargine or NPH insulin
Drugs used	Insulin glargine once daily, NPH insulin once or twice daily, doses depending on fasting plasma glucose (FPG) levels
Patients	534 well-controlled patients with type 1 diabetes, with HbA_{1c} levels ≤12.0%
Outcomes	Mean change from baseline in HbA_{1c} and capillary FPG, median change from baseline in FPG, incidence of hypoglycaemia with a blood glucose level <2.0 mmol/L
Analysis	Intention to treat, last observation carried forward. Changes in HbA_{1c} and FPG values assessed with ANCOVA models
Follow-up	28 weeks

Results

Glycaemic control (change from baseline to endpoint)			
	Insulin glargine	NPH	P compared with baseline
HbA$_{1c}$, %	-0.16	-0.21	0.4408
Capillary FBG (mmol/L)	-1.12	-0.94	0.3546
FPG (mmol/L)	-1.67	-0.33	0.0145
Percentage of patients reporting at least one episode of hypoglycaemia and number of episodes per 100 patient-years			
	All hypoglycaemia	Severe hypoglycaemia	Nocturnal hypoglycaemia
Insulin glargine			
Subjects, %	39.9	1.9	18.2
Episodes (per 100 patient-years)	200.5	7.9	65.1
NPH insulin			
Patients, %	49.2*	5.6	27.1*
Episodes (per 100 patient-years)	345.4	16.7	101.2
*P<0.05 versus insulin glargine			

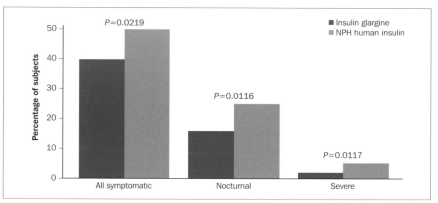

Figure 57. Percentages of patients reporting at least one episode of symptomatic, nocturnal or severe hypoglycaemia confirmed by a blood glucose level <2.0 mmol/L. Reproduced with permission from the American Diabetes Association.

Commentary

The potential advantages of insulin glargine over traditional basal insulin such as NPH and ultralente are seen by its flattened time-action profile, full 24-hour profile and once-daily dosing. The expectation was that this insulin would produce a more physiological insulin profile when used in patients with type 1 or type 2 diabetes.

Indeed, studies in type 1 diabetes have shown no difference from standard formulations from the point of view of HbA$_{1c}$, but reduced risk of nocturnal hypoglycaemia and lower FPG.

This study by Ratner et al compared insulin glargine with NPH insulin in patients with type 2 diabetes who had previously been treated with multiple daily injections of NPH insulin and regular insulin. Glargine was found to be safe and well tolerated, with benefits as described above, including lower fasting glucose and reduced episodes of hypoglycaemia.

Insulin glargine has since been granted a licence for use in both type 1 and type 2 diabetes. It is now a commonly used insulin as part of a basal bolus regimen in type 1 diabetes, and in combination with oral agents or regular insulin in type 2 diabetes.

Effects of metformin in patients with poorly controlled, insulin-treated type 2 diabetes mellitus

What does this trial tell us?

➤ The addition of metformin to insulin therapy results in HbA_{1c} concentrations 10% lower than those achieved with insulin alone

➤ The improvement in glycaemic control occurred with 29% less insulin and without significant weight gain

➤ The Results indicate that metformin is an effective adjunct to insulin in type 2 diabetes

Authors	Avilés-Santa L, Sinding J, Raskin P
Reference	*Ann Intern Med* 1999;**131**:182–8
Objective	To evaluate the efficacy of metformin in combination with insulin in type 2 diabetes that is poorly controlled with insulin alone
Methodology	Randomised, double-blind, placebo-controlled trial of metformin or placebo in addition to insulin
Drugs used	Insulin, dose adjusted according to fasting blood glucose; metformin 1.5–2.0 g/day
Patients	43 patients with poorly controlled type 2 diabetes who were receiving insulin therapy
Outcomes	Primary endpoints were glycaemic control and insulin dose requirements. Secondary endpoints included body weight and blood pressure changes
Analysis	Intention to treat
Follow-up	24 weeks

Results

Characteristic	Metformin group		Placebo group	
	Baseline (mean)	Change from baseline (mean)	Baseline (mean)	Change from baseline (mean)
Body weight (kg)	103.9	0.5	106.6	3.2 ($P<0.01$)
Insulin dose (U/day)	96.2	−4.5	96.9	22.8 ($P<0.001$)
Fasting plasma glucose (mg/dL)	197.2	−63.1	218.5 ($P<0.001$)	−64.8 ($P<0.001$)
HbA$_{1c}$ level	9.0%	−2.5 percentage points ($P<0.001$)	9.1%	−1.6 percentage points ($P<0.001$)

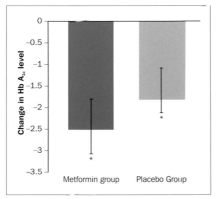

Figure 58. Change in HbA$_{1c}$ level from baseline to 24 weeks. Error bars represent the standard deviation. *$P<0.001$ compared with baseline. Reproduced with permission from the American College of Physicians–American Society of Internal Medicine.

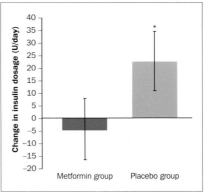

Figure 59. Change in daily insulin dose from baseline to 24 weeks. Error bars represent the standard deviation. *$P<0.001$ compared with baseline. Reproduced with permission from the American College of Physicians–American Society of Internal Medicine.

Commentary

Type 2 diabetes is a progressive disease, and the majority of patients will eventually require insulin to achieve adequate glycaemic control. The downside of this is the usual requirement for large doses of insulin, weight gain and increased risk of hypoglycaemia. The combination of insulin with oral agents has received much attention as a means of allowing tightened diabetic control with less insulin usage and a reduced risk of treatment-related side effects. This is particularly so for metformin combinations. In this study, the combination of metformin with insulin resulted in a further improvement in HbA_{1c}, reduced the insulin dose and caused no significant weight gain.

As a result of this and other studies, the combination of insulin with metformin is now commonly used as a treatment in the management of type 2 diabetes.

Glycemic control with diet, sulfonylurea, metformin, or insulin in patients with type 2 diabetes mellitus. Progressive requirement for multiple therapies (UKPDS 49)

What does this trial tell us?

➤ Each therapeutic agent, as monotherapy, initially achieves satisfactory glycaemic control compared with diet alone

➤ Glycaemic control with monotherapy deteriorates progressively, even within 3 years

➤ Most patients need multiple therapies to maintain satisfactory glycaemic control

---

Authors	Turner, RC, Cull CA, Frighi V, Holman RR, for the UK Prospective Diabetes Study (UKPDS) Group
Reference	*JAMA* 1999;281:2005–12
Objective	To assess how often diet, insulin, sulphonylurea or metformin, as monotherapies, can achieve satisfactory glycaemic control
Methodology	Randomised controlled trial in 15 diabetes outpatient clinics
Drugs used	Insulin, sulphonylurea, chlorpropamide and glyburide; doses according to fasting plasma glucose (FPG) and HbA_{1c} levels
Patients	4,075 patients, aged 25–65 years, newly diagnosed with type 2 diabetes
Outcomes	FPG and HbA_{1c} levels, and the proportion of patients who achieved target levels of HbA_{1c} <7.0% or FPG <7.8 mmol/L at 3, 6 or 9 years
Analysis	Intention to treat. Logistic regression analysis to detect factors that could have predicted failure to attain target levels. Analysis to assess requirement for multiple therapies
Follow-up	9 years

Results

Proportions of patients who attained goals (%), normal and overweight patients combined				
Therapy	HbA₁c<7.0%		FPG <7.8 mmol/L	
	3 years	9 years	3 years	9 years
Diet	25	9	19	8
Insulin	47	28	52	42
Chlorpropamide	53	28	51	28
Glyburide	47	20	41	20
Sulphonylurea	50	24	46	24

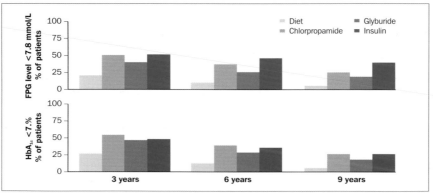

Figure 60. Proportions of patients who received monotherapy and achieved control targets after 3, 6 and 9 years. FPG: fasting plasma glucose. Reproduced with permission from the American Medical Association.

Commentary

This study has profoundly important practical implications. The authors clearly showed that type 2 diabetes is a progressive disease and that although most patients will initially manage on a controlled diet or diet plus a monotherapy regimen, over time, the great majority will require more intensive treatment with multiple agents.

Many studies have shown evidence of under-treatment of type 2 diabetes, with an extremely protracted time to initiation of the first oral agent, and then to the second or even third oral agent followed by insulin. The result is years of poor control and late usage of therapies that would have been more appropriate much earlier in the disease process. The clear message is that, over time, the great majority of type 2 diabetic patients will require combination treatment. This should not be delayed as consequent poor control is a reason for a significantly increased risk of vascular complications.

Effect of metformin and rosiglitazone combination therapy in patients with type 2 diabetes mellitus. A randomized controlled trial

What does this trial tell us?

➤ Combination treatment with once-daily metformin–rosiglitazone improves glycaemic control, insulin sensitivity and beta-cell function more effectively than metformin alone

➤ The combination is safe and well tolerated

Authors	Fonseca V, Rosenstock J, Patwardhan R, Salzman A
Reference	*JAMA* 2000;283:1695–702
Objective	To investigate the efficacy of metformin–rosiglitazone therapy in patients whose type 2 diabetes is inadequately controlled with metformin alone
Methodology	Randomised, double-blind, placebo-controlled, 36-centre trial of metformin–rosiglitazone therapy versus metformin
Drugs used	Metformin 2.5 g/day plus placebo, metformin 2.5 g/day plus rosiglitazone 4 mg/day, or metformin 2.5 g/day plus rosiglitazone 8 mg/day
Patients	348 patients, aged 40–80 years, with mean HbA_{1c} 8.8%, mean fasting plasma glucose 12.0 mmol/L and mean body mass index 30.1 kg/m^2
Outcomes	HbA_{1c} levels, fasting plasma glucose levels, insulin sensitivity, beta-cell function
Analysis	Intention to treat
Follow-up	26 weeks

127

Results

Changes from baseline at 26 weeks			
Treatment	Metformin + placebo	Metformin + rosiglitazone 4 mg/day	Metformin + rosiglitazone 8 mg/day
Mean change in HbA$_{1c}$ (%)	+0.45 (P<0.0001)	−0.56 (P<0.001)	−0.78 (P<0.001)
Mean change in fasting plasma glucose (mg/dL)	+5.9 (P<0.18)	−33.0 (P<0.001)	−48.4 (P<0.001)

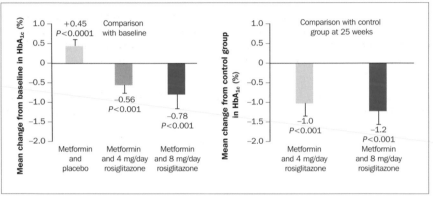

Figure 61. Changes in HbA$_{1c}$ levels at week 26 in patients on metformin and rosiglitazone compared with metformin alone. Reproduced with permission from the American Medical Association.

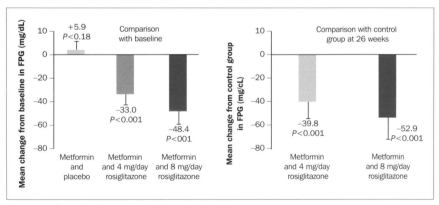

Figure 62. Changes in fasting plasma glucose concentrations at week 26 in patients on metformin and rosiglitazone compared with metformin alone. FPG: fasting plasma glucose. Reproduced with permission from the American Medical Association.

Commentary

Although sulphonylureas and biguanides have been around for 50 years, the thiazolidines (glitazones) represent one of several classes of agents that have appeared in recent years to treat diabetes. This study was the first to report on the efficacy of rosiglitazone in combination with metformin. Glitazones act on an intranuclear hormone receptor (peroxisome proliferator-activated receptor gamma) to produce effects on carbohydrate and lipid metabolism similar to those that occur when insulin combines with its receptor. These agents therefore have an insulin-sparing effect, improving insulin sensitivity and thereby reducing insulin resistance.

Metformin is thought to have positive effects on insulin sensitivity by different mechanisms. The combination of metformin and rosiglitazone therefore seemed to have a good theoretical base. Indeed, in this study it was associated with significant reductions in HbA_{1c} and fasting plasma glucose, and improvements in insulin sensitivity and beta-cell function.

Glitazones have a rather limited licence in Europe, although their use is much wider in the US. Various important studies are ongoing to determine whether these agents might be particularly useful in preserving long-term glycaemic control and (perhaps through their effects on insulin resistance) reducing cardiovascular risk.

Inhaled human insulin treatment in patients with type 2 diabetes mellitus

What does this trial tell us?

➤ In patients with type 2 diabetes requiring improved glycaemic control, pulmonary delivery of insulin is well tolerated and demonstrates no adverse pulmonary effects

Authors	Cefalu WT, Skyler JS, Kourides IA, et al, for the Inhaled Insulin Study Group
Reference	*Ann Intern Med* 2001;134:203–7
Objective	To assess the efficacy and safety of pulmonary delivery of insulin in patients with type 2 diabetes who require insulin
Methodology	Randomised, open-label study of insulin delivered by a mechanical inhaler, consisting of a screening visit, a 4-week lead-in phase and a 12-week treatment phase
Drugs used	Inhaled insulin 1 mg/day or 3 mg/day during treatment phase, plus ultralente insulin daily at bedtime as the sole long-acting insulin
Patients	26 patients with type 2 diabetes, aged 35–65 years, on stable insulin schedules
Outcomes	Glycaemic control (HbA_{1c}), pulmonary function tests, adverse events
Analysis	Efficacy assessed by 12-week change in HbA_{1c} level from baseline
Follow-up	3 months

Results

Outcome	Comment
HbA_{1c} level	Decreased significantly from mean 8.67% at baseline to mean 7.96% at 12 weeks (see **Figure 32**)
Hypoglycaemic events	0.83 mild–moderate events per month; 39 in the first 4 weeks, 22 in the last 8 weeks
Adverse events	No severe events recorded
Pulmonary function	No significant changes from baseline in spirometry results, lung volume, diffusion capacity or oxygen saturation

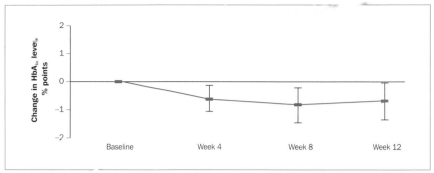

Figure 63. Change in mean HbA$_{1c}$ level during the 12-week treatment phase in type 2 diabetic patients receiving inhaled insulin therapy. Error bars represent 1 standard deviation. Reproduced with permission from the American College of Physicians–American Society of Internal Medicine.

Commentary

Alternative methods of insulin delivery have been sought for many decades. Indeed, the first report on inhaling insulin to treat diabetes goes back to the 1920s. It is only in recent years, however, that the technology has developed to allow this to become a practical possibility. In this study, the authors showed pulmonary delivery of insulin to be associated with improved glycaemic control in patients with type 2 diabetes. There appeared to be no adverse pulmonary effects.

Since then, a range of large-scale studies have been performed in both type 1 and type 2 diabetes. Compared with standard regular injectable insulin, these have basically shown equivalence of HbA$_{1c}$, (probably) no significant difference in risk of hypoglycaemia and high patient satisfaction.

Efficacy of inhaled human insulin in type 1 diabetes mellitus: a randomised proof-of-concept study

What does this trial tell us?

➤ Preprandial insulin given by inhalation achieves good glycaemic control in patients with insulin-deficient type 1 diabetes

➤ Inhaled insulin does not affect pulmonary function or cause adverse events

➤ Inhaled insulin may be a less invasive alternative to insulin injections

Authors	Skyler JS, Cefalu WT, Kourides IA, et al, for the Inhaled Insulin Phase II Study Group
Reference	*Lancet* 2001;357:331–5
Objective	To investigate the safety and efficacy of intrapulmonary delivery of insulin
Methodology	Open-label, proof-of-concept, parallel-group, randomised trial of inhaled preprandial insulin plus bedtime subcutaneous ultralente insulin versus usual subcutaneous insulin regimen
Drugs used	Inhaled insulin 1 mg or 3 mg by aerosol three times daily, ultralente insulin daily at bedtime, both depending on glucose monitoring results; insulin injections according to usual dose
Patients	73 patients with type 1 diabetes on a stable insulin schedule
Outcomes	The primary endpoint was change in HbA_{1c} level. Secondary endpoints were fasting and postprandial glucose response to a mixed meal, hypoglycaemia frequency and severity, pulmonary function and patient satisfaction
Analysis	Intention to treat. Change in HbA_{1c} levels was analysed by use of an analysis of covariance model
Follow-up	12 weeks

Results

Outcome	Comment			
HbA$_{1c}$ levels, fasting and postprandial glucose	Changes similar or indistinguishable between inhaled and and subcutaneous groups (see **Figures 39 and 40**)			
Pulmonary function	Stable throughout study period. No significant difference in pulmonary function tests between groups			
Adverse events	No major adverse events			
Outcome	Inhaled insulin		Subcutaneous insulin	
	Mild–moderate	Severe	Mild–moderate	Severe
Hypoglycaemia				
Patients with hypoglycaemia, n (%)	33 (94.3%)	5 (14.3%)	31 (83.8%)	5 (13.5%)
Episodes, n	550	8	547	10
Episodes per patient-month	5.5	0.08	5.3	0.10

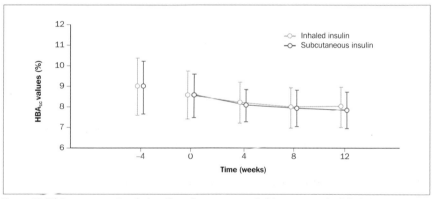

Figure 64. HbA$_{1c}$ concentration during 12-week treatment period (mean ± standard deviation). Reproduced with permission from *The Lancet*.

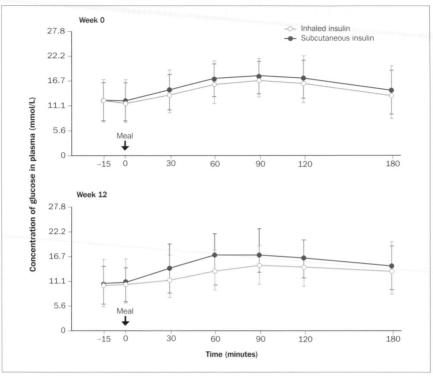

Figure 65. Plasma glucose concentration in response to a test meal at baseline and after 12 weeks of treatment (mean ± standard deviation). Reproduced with permission from *The Lancet*.

Commentary

The concept of alternative routes of insulin delivery, other than injections, has been around for many years. It is only recently, however, that technology has progressed sufficiently to make this a practical proposition.

In this study, inhaled preprandial insulin plus subcutaneous basal insulin was compared with a usual insulin regimen. Inhaled preprandial insulin achieved as good glycaemic control as that given by injection, and there appeared to be no significant adverse effects on pulmonary function. This was a seminal proof-of-concept study that has led to many other studies of inhaled insulin.

Training in flexible, intensive insulin management to enable dietary freedom in people with type 1 diabetes: Dose Adjustment for Normal Eating (DAFNE) randomised controlled trial

What does this trial tell us?

➤ Dietary skills training improves quality of life (QOL) and glycaemic control in patients with type 1 diabetes, without increasing cardiovascular or hypoglycaemic risk

➤ This approach may enable more patients to adopt intensive insulin treatment

Authors	Dose Adjustment for Normal Eating (DAFNE) Study Group
Reference	*BMJ* 2002;325:746–59
Objective	To evaluate whether a course teaching flexible insulin treatment that combines dietary freedom and insulin adjustment can improve glycaemic control and QOL in type 1 diabetes
Methodology	Randomised controlled trial comparing immediate attendance at a DAFNE course with attendance after 6 months on waiting list
Drugs used	Insulin as required, principally by matching to desired carbohydrate intake
Patients	169 adults with type 1 diabetes, moderate or poor glycaemic control (HbA$_{1c}$ 7.5–12%) and >2 years' duration of diabetes without advanced complications
Outcomes	HbA$_{1c}$, severe hypoglycaemia, impact of diabetes on QOL (Audit of Diabetes Dependent Quality of Life [ADDQoL])
Analysis	6-month outcomes compared using unpaired *t* tests; hypoglycaemia at 6 and 12 months compared using chi-squared tests
Follow-up	1 year

Results

Mean differences between immediate DAFNE and delayed DAFNE groups at 6 months				
Group	HbA$_{1c}$, % (SD)	Proportion experiencing severe hypoglycaemia, n (%)	ADDQoL score	
			Weighted impact of diabetes on 'freedom to eat as I wish'	Average weighted impact of diabetes on QOL
Immediate DAFNE				
Baseline	9.4 (1.2)	15/68 (22)	−4.8	−2.0
6 months	8.4 (1.2)	12/67 (18)	−1.8	−1.6
Delayed DAFNE				
Baseline	9.3 (1.1)	8/72 (11)	−4.0	−1.9
6 months	9.4 (1.3)	11/72 (15)	−4.0	−1.9
Difference between groups at 6 months				
Mean	1.0	–	2.2	0.4
P values	<0.0001	0.68	<0.0001	<0.01

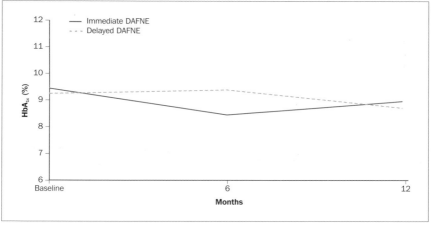

Figure 66. Glycaemic control in immediate and delayed DAFNE (Dose Adjustment For Normal Eating) groups. Reproduced with permission from BMJ Publishing.

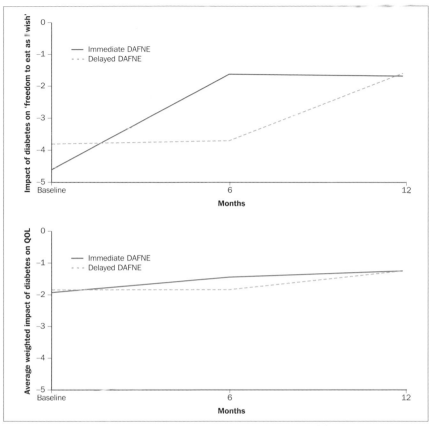

Figure 67. Reported impact of diabetes on (**top**) 'freedom to act as I wish' and (**bottom**) average weighted impact of diabetes on quality of life. DAFNE: Dose Adjustment For Normal Eating; QOL: quality of life. Reproduced with permission from BMJ Publishing.

Commentary

Historically, management of type 1 diabetes has involved balancing food intake, exercise and insulin dose. Many diabetic patients and their carers feel that this leads to reduced treatment satisfaction and QOL. The DAFNE approach has been applied to patients receiving intensified insulin regimens. This approach aims to combine dietary freedom with insulin adjustment to improve treatment satisfaction and QOL.

The principal findings from this study included the observation that training and flexibility in diet and lifestyle improved QOL and glycaemic control in people with type 1 diabetes, without increasing vascular risk factors or risk of hypoglycaemia. This is an area of intense interest, with major practical implications. More studies are being performed to see how widely applicable this methodology might be.

Lifestyle intervention by group care prevents deterioration of type 2 diabetes: a 4-year randomized controlled clinical trial

What does this trial tell us?

➤ Group care by systematic education is cost-effective in preventing deterioration of metabolic control and quality of life in type 2 diabetes

➤ The treatment is feasible in an ordinary diabetes clinic

Authors	Trento M, Passera P, Bajardi M, et al
Reference	*Diabetologia* 2002;45:1231–9
Objective	To test a model of systematic group education in patients with type 2 diabetes
Methodology	Randomised controlled trial of systemic group education compared with individual consultations and education (controls)
Drugs used	Patients' usual hypoglycaemic agents
Patients	56 patients, aged 35–78 years, with non-insulin-treated type 2 diabetes and 56 control patients
Outcomes	Primary endpoints included body weight, fasting blood glucose, HbA_{1c} and blood lipids, plus health behaviour and quality of life according to standardised scales. Secondary endpoints included diabetic retinopathy, hypoglycaemic medication and blood pressure
Analysis	Intention to treat
Follow-up	51.2 ± 2 months

Results

Knowledge of diabetes, health behaviours and quality of life at baseline and at 4 years (means on standardised scales)						
	Group care patients			Control patients		
	Baseline	4 years	Difference	Baseline	4 years	Difference
Knowledge of diabetes	14.9	27.1	+12.2*	20.4	17.2	–3.2**
Health behaviours	11.0	16.5	+5.4*	12.3	10.2	–2.1*
Quality of life	67.6	44.0	–23.6*	70.5	89.8	+19.2*
*P<0.001, **P<0.05						
Cost-effectiveness: Each point gained in quality of life was obtained with an expenditure of only US$2.12						

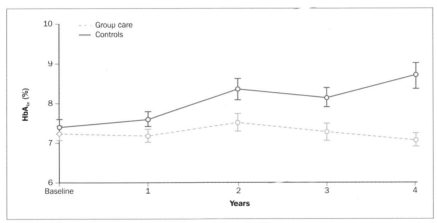

Figure 68. HbA₁c in group care patients and controls from baseline to year 4. Valves are means ± standard errors. Reproduced with permission from Springer-Verlag.

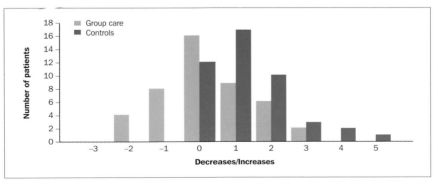

Figure 69. Changes in hypoglycaemic medication in group care patients and controls from baseline to year 4 (for differences between groups, *P*<0.001). Reproduced with permission from Springer-Verlag.

Commentary

Given the great increase in the numbers of patients with type 2 diabetes, this was a timely study. Trento et al looked at the effectiveness of systematic group education compared with individual consultations and education for patients with type 2 diabetes. They found group care to be cost-effective in preventing deterioration of metabolic control and quality of life in type 2 diabetes, and found the treatment to be feasible in an ordinary diabetes clinic.

Many diabetes services now utilise this methodology. It is not ideal for all patients, but it is certainly a management option for the majority.

Sulfonylurea inadequacy. Efficacy of addition of insulin over 6 years in patients with type 2 diabetes in the UK Prospective Diabetes Study (UKPDS 57)

What does this trial tell us?

➤ Early addition of insulin when maximal sulphonylurea treatment is inadequate can significantly improve glycaemic control

➤ The combination does not promote weight gain or increase the risk of hypoglycaemia

Authors	Wright A, Burden ACF, Paisey RB, et al, for the UKPDS Group
Reference	*Diabetes Care* 2002;25:330–6
Objective	To evaluate the efficacy of adding insulin when maximal sulphonylurea dose is inadequate for glycaemic control in type 2 diabetes
Methodology	Randomised controlled study comparing conventional glucose control (primarily with diet), an intensive policy with insulin alone and addition of insulin to patients receiving sulphonylurea if fasting plasma glucose (FPG) remained >6.0 mmol/L despite maximum sulphonylurea dose
Drugs used	Insulin, chlorpropamide, glipizide; sulphonylurea doses according to fasting blood glucose
Patients	826 patients, mean age 52 years, with newly diagnosed type 2 diabetes
Outcomes	Glycaemic control (HbA$_{1c}$), hypoglycaemia, body weight
Analysis	Intention to treat, apart from occurrence of hypoglycaemia
Follow-up	6 years

Results

Glycaemic control over 6 years and proportion of patients experiencing major hypoglycaemic episodes					
	HbA$_{1c}$			Major hypoglycaemic episodes	
Allocation	% Median	P versus conventional glucose control	P versus insulin alone	% Patients per annum	P versus insulin alone
Conventional glucose control	7.6			0	
Intensive glucose control					
Insulin alone	7.1	<0.00001		3.4	
Sulphonylurea (± insulin)	6.6	<0.00001	0.0066	1.6	0.0033
Chlorpropamide (± insulin)	6.6	<0.00001	0.010	1.8	0.044
Glipizide (± insulin)	6.7	0.00001	0.048	1.4	0.0076

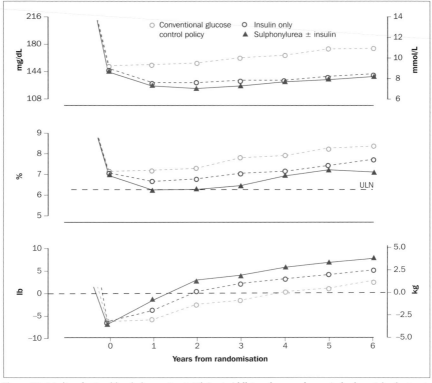

Figure 70. Median fasting blood glucose (**top**), HbA$_{1c}$ (**middle**) and mean change in body weight (**bottom**) over a 6-year follow-up. ULN: upper limit of normal. Reproduced with permission from the American Diabetes Association.

Commentary

Although an insulin/metformin combination is very commonly used in the management of type 2 diabetes, an insulin/sulphonylurea combination has, until recently, been much less common. This study, again relating to the UKPDS programme, evaluated the efficacy of adding insulin when the maximum sulphonylurea dose is inadequate to achieve glycaemic control in type 2 diabetes. The authors found that early addition of insulin to the maximum sulphonylurea therapy significantly improved glycaemic control. This was not associated with weight gain or an increased risk of hypoglycaemia.

The insulin/metformin combination remains a very common treatment for type 2 diabetes and, to date, there is less convincing evidence for the insulin/sulphonylurea combination. However, this is increasingly being recognised as a management option. There is the further possibility of using an insulin/metformin/sulphonylurea combination in the management of type 2 diabetes.

Combination of insulin and metformin in the treatment of type 2 diabetes

What does this trial tell us?

➤ In patients with type 2 diabetes intensively treated with insulin, the addition of metformin results in significantly improved glycaemic control

➤ Insulin requirements and weight gain are less in patients treated with the combination of insulin and metformin

Authors	Wulffelé MG, Kooy A, Lehert P, et al
Reference	*Diabetes Care* 2002;25:2133–40
Objective	To investigate the effects of metformin in type 2 diabetic patients intensively treated with insulin
Methodology	Randomised controlled, double-blind trial of insulin plus either placebo or metformin
Drugs used	Insulin, metformin; dose depending on self-administered glucose level testing
Patients	390 patients with type 2 diabetes treated at entry, either exclusively with insulin or with insulin plus metformin
Outcomes	Primary endpoints were glycaemic control (HbA$_{1c}$) and daily insulin requirement. Secondary endpoints were body mass index (BMI), body weight, plasma cholesterol, plasma triglycerides and blood pressure
Analysis	Intention to treat
Follow-up	16-week short-term phase, 48-month long-term phase

Results

Mean changes in HbA$_{1c}$, insulin requirement, body weight and BMI at 16 weeks							
	Baseline		Follow-up		Change		
Outcome parameter	Placebo	Metformin	Placebo	Metformin	Placebo	Metformin	P value
HbA$_{1c}$ (% Hb)	7.88	7.86	7.61	6.94	−0.27	−0.91	<0.0001
Daily dose of insulin (IU/day)	69.9	71	71.3	63.8	1.4	−7.2	<0.0001
Body weight (kg)	86.2	85.6	87.4	85.1	1.2	−0.4	<0.0001
BMI (kg/m^2)	29.5	29.9	30	29.7	0.4	−0.2	0.001

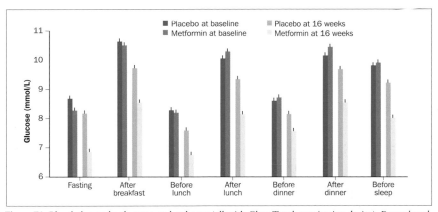

Figure 71. Blood glucose levels measured at home (all with GlucoTouch monitoring device). Reproduced with permission from the American Diabetes Association.

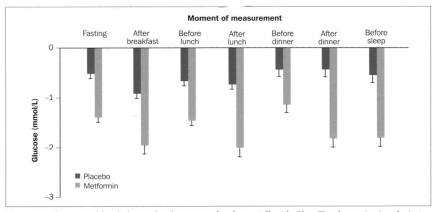

Figure 72. Changes in blood glucose levels measured at home (all with GlucoTouch monitoring device). Reproduced with permission from the American Diabetes Association.

Commentary

This trial emphasises that, even in patients with type 2 diabetes intensively treated with insulin, the addition of the oral anti-diabetic agent metformin will result in even better control, with the likelihood of a reduction in insulin requirement and less weight gain. Until recently, the use of insulin/oral anti-diabetic combinations has not been a popular approach in many countries. This study, and others, has emphasised the benefits of such an approach and suggests that unless there is a contraindication or tolerability problem, metformin should be added to the management regimen of all patients with type 2 diabetes who require some kind of pharmacotherapy. This is further emphasised by the cardiovascular protective benefits demonstrated by the UKPDS.

Conclusions

Conclusions

This book is one author's attempt to pick out clinical trials relevant to diabetes – those that I believe have had a major impact on diabetes management. They are a tribute to the hard work, dedication and enthusiasm of thousands of investigators worldwide.

I have deliberately not included the many landmark studies of a more basic scientific nature, although these have greatly aided our understanding of the pathogenesis of diabetes and its long term complications. Apologies to the many excellent researchers in these areas.

A significant proportion, but by no means all, of these studies come from the stable of the UK Prospective Diabetes Study. This is a great tribute to one man, Robert Turner, who originally conceived the idea for this work and brought it to fruition over 20 years later. Robert saw UKPDS come to a successful end, and I was privileged to be present at the European Association for the Study of Diabetes meeting in Barcelona in 1998 when the first results were presented to a packed audience.

Unfortunately, Robert died soon after completion of this project and I would very much like to dedicate this book to his memory. There have, of course, been many other extremely important trials not related to UKPDS, and they are also a great tribute to the many researchers involved. Because of their work we now have a real evidence base on which to work and to improve the lot of our patients.

Anthony Barnett

Index